D1631152

# Biocompatibility Assessment of Medical Devices and Materials

# Wiley Series in Biomaterials Science and Engineering

Commissioned in the UK on behalf of John Wiley & Sons, Ltd by Medi-Tech Publications, Storrington, West Sussex RH20 4HH, UK

Series Advisors

**Robin N. Stephens**
AVE (UK) Limited, Burgess Hill, UK

**Julian H. Braybrook**
Laboratory of the Government Chemist, London, UK

**Patrick M. Maloney**
CellPro Inc, Bothell, Washington, USA

Providing readers with comprehensive, authoritative and timely information in this fast-developing area of research and biomedical technological advancement, this series encompasses topics in biomaterials science and engineering including the structure and function of materials and devices, their individual actions and interactions, and practical and clinical applications.

Books in the *Wiley Series in Biomaterials Science and Engineering* are designed to help stimulate further developments in biomaterials science and engineering by disseminating up-to-the-minute, quality information to academic and industrial research and development scientists employed in all areas of the medical, biomedical and bioengineering sciences, whether in medical device R&D, pharmaceutical and pharmacological research or materials science, and to clinical specialists in posthesis and surgery.

## RECENT TITLES IN THE SERIES

*Biosensors in the Body, Continuous in vivo Monitoring*
Edited by David M. Fraser (0-471-96707-6)

*Biocompatibility Assessment of Medical Devices and Materials*
Edited by Julian H. Braybrook (0-471-96597-9)

## FORTHCOMING TITLES IN THE SERIES

*Design Engineering of Biomaterials for Medical Devices*
David M. Hill (0-471-96708-4)

*Metals as Biomaterials*
Edited by J. Helsen and J. Breme (0-471-96935-4)

*Computer Technology in Biomaterials Science and Engineering*
Edited by J. Vander Sloten (0-471-97602-4)

# Biocompatibility Assessment of Medical Devices and Materials

Edited by

## Julian H. Braybrook
London, United Kingdom

JOHN WILEY & SONS
Chichester · New York · Weinheim · Brisbane · Toronto · Singapore

Copyright © 1997 by John Wiley & Sons Ltd,
Baffins Lane, Chichester,
West Sussex PO19 1UD, England

National　　01243 779777
International (+44) 1243 779777
e-mail (for orders and customer service enquiries): cs-books@wiley.co.uk
Visit our Home Page on http://www.wiley.co.uk
or http://www.wiley.com

*Other Wiley Editorial Offices*

John Wiley & Sons, Inc., 605 Third Avenue,
New York, NY 10158-0012, USA

VCH Verlagsgesellschaft mbh, Pappelallee 3,
D-69469 Weinheim, Germany

Jacaranda Wiley Ltd, 33 Park Road, Milton,
Queensland 4064, Australia

John Wiley & Sons (Asia) Pte Ltd, 2 Clementi Loop #02-01,
Jin Xing Distripark, Singapore 129809

John Wiley & Sons (Canada) Ltd, 22 Worcester Road,
Rexdale, Ontario M9W 1LI, Canada

*Library of Congress Cataloging-in-Publication Data*

Biocompatibility assessment of medical devices and materials / edited by Julian H. Braybrook.
　　p.　cm. – (Biomaterials science and engineering)
　　Includes bibliographical references and index.
　　ISBN 0-471-96597-9
　　1. Biomedical materials—Biocompatibility—Testing.　2. Biomedical materials— Standards.
　　I. Braybrook, Julian.　II. Series.
　　[DNLM: 1. Biocompatible Materials.　2. Equipment and Supplies.
　　3. Materials Testing.　QT 37 B613 1997]
　　R857.M3B524　1997
　　610'.28—dc21
　　DNLM/DLC
　　for Library of Congress
　　　　　　　　　　　　　　　　　　　　　　　　　　　96–29705
　　　　　　　　　　　　　　　　　　　　　　　　　　　CIP

*British Library Cataloguing in Publication Data*

A catalogue record for this book is available from the British Library

ISBN 0-471-96597-9

Typeset in 10/12pt Times from the author's disks by Vision Typesetting, Manchester
Printed and bound in Great Britain by Biddles Ltd, Guildford
This book is printed on acid-free paper responsibly manufactured from sustainable forestation,
for which at least two trees are planted for each one used for paper production.

# Contents

# List of Contributors

JAMES ANDERSON

*Institute of Pathology, Case Western Reserve University School of Clinical Medicine, University Hospitals of Cleveland, 2085 Adelbert Road, Cleveland OH 44106-4907, USA*
*Professor of Pathology at Case Western Reserve University and Convenor of ISO/TC 194 WG1 (Systemic approach to biological evaluation and terminology)*

JULIAN BRAYBROOK

*Laboratory of the Government Chemist (LGC), Queens Road, Teddington, Middlesex TW11 0LY, UK*
*Business Manager at LGC, Special biomaterials consultant to Medi-Tech Publications, and European project leader for CEN/TC 206 to ISO/TC 194 WG12 (Sample preparation and reference materials)*

JAGDISH BUTANY

*General Division, Department of Pathology, The Toronto Hospital and University of Toronto, 200 Elizabeth Street, Toronto, Ontario M5G 2C4, Canada*
*Associate Professor at the University of Toronto*

MARTYN DAVIES

*Department of Pharmaceutical Sciences, The University of Nottingham, University Park, Nottingham NG7 2RD, UK*
*Professor of Biomedical Surface Chemistry at the University of Nottingham*

VICTOR DORMAN-SMITH

*Scientific Affairs, Abbott Ireland, Sligo, Ireland*
*Scientific Affairs Manager at Abbott*

JAN-WILLEM DORPEMA

*Laboratory for Medicines and Medical Devices,
Rijksinstituut voor Volksgezondheid en Milieu
(RIVM), Antonie van Leeuwenhoeklaan 9,
PO Box 1, 3720 Bilthoven, The Netherlands
Head of Laboratory for Medicines and Medical
Devices at RIVM, and Chairman of CEN/TC 206
(Biological evaluation of medical and dental
materials and devices)*

ROSY ELOY

*Biomatech, Z.I.de l'Islon, Rue Pasteur, 38760
Chasse-sur-Rhone, France
Director of Biomatech*

DAVID GOTT

*Medical Devices Agency, Department of Health,
14 Russell Square, London WC1B 5EP, UK
Toxicologist at the Medical Devices Agency*

MARIE-FRANÇOISE
HARMAND

*Laboratoire d'Evaluation des Matériels
Implantables (LEMI), Technopole Montesquieu,
33650 Martillac, France
Scientific Director at LEMI, Lecturer at
INSERM U443 at the University of Bordeaux II,
and Convenor of ISO/TC 194 WG5
(Cytotoxicity)*

MARJA KUIJPERS

*Laboratory for Medicines and Medical Devices,
Rijksinstituut voor Volksgezondheid en Milieu
(RIVM), Antonie van Leeuwenhoeklaan 9, PO
Box 1, 3720 Bilthoven, The Netherlands
Laboratory of Medicines and Medical Devices at
RIVM, and Secretary of CEN/TC 206 (Biological
evaluation of medical and dental materials and
devices)*

DON MARLOWE

*Office of Science and Technology, US Food and
Drug Administration (FDA), Center for Devices
for Radiological Health, 9200 Corporate
Boulevard (HFZ-100), Rockville MD 20850, USA
Director of Office of Science and Technology at
FDA, and Convenor of ISO/TC 194 WG 12
(Sample preparation and reference materials)*

C. J. ROBERTS

*Department of Pharmaceutical Sciences, The University of Nottingham, University Park, Nottingham NG7 2RD, UK*

S. J. B. TENDLER

*Department of Pharmaceutical Sciences, The University of Nottingham, University Park, Nottingham NG7 2RD, UK*

JEREMY TINKLER

*Medical Devices Agency, Department of Health, 14 Russell Square, London WC1B 5EP, UK Toxicologist at the Medical Devices Agency, and Convenor of CEN/BTS3 WG1 Task Force on Toxicological Risk Analysis*

N. WEILL

*Biomatech, Z.I. de l'Islon, Rue Pasteur, 38760 Chasse-sur-Rhône, France*

P. M. WILLIAMS

*Department of Pharmaceutical Sciences, The University of Nottingham, University Park, Nottingham NG7 2RD, UK*

# Preface

As medical procedures become more sophisticated and the application of novel materials as prostheses or in medical devices receives increasing interest, the market for biocompatible materials continues to grow rapidly. However, to sustain such growth, the evaluation and subsequent comparison of the biocompatibility of materials (i.e. their ability to perform with an appropriate host response in a specific application) requires tests that are fully appropriate, that is, they must increasingly provide solutions to understanding the host response and the issues pertaining to it. It is this complexity which restricts the accuracy and reliability of existing test methodology. Indeed it is becoming all the more evident that severe limitations in the function and/or biocompatibility of a number of existing prostheses may still exist. Both the healthcare industry and patients alike are more discerning and aware of the potential difficulties. Thus it is going to take a change of viewpoint and the systematic evaluation of desired biological, chemical and engineering requirements to provide the infrastructure to allow the derivation of materials with long-term clinical acceptance, that is, true biocompatibility.

It was this dilemma which, several years ago, brought about the acknowledgement by the biomaterials industry that the adoption of many medical materials and devices had been on a trial-and-error off-the-shelf basis and that the valuable traditional approach of sole reliance on the skill and experience of specialist scientists now required support from multidisciplinary teams using an agreed range of methodologies, the accreditation of participating test laboratories, and the adoption of quality protocols supported by certified reference materials, CRMs. This new philosophy dovetailed with the overall initiative aiming to encourage all laboratories to demonstrate the validity of analytical measurement (VAM) and thereby facilitate the mutual recognition of data and their subsequent understanding. Nevertheless, despite odd pockets of activity, there has until recently been little coordinated international effort to bring these protocols and materials together. It may be that in many circles this viewpoint has been counted upon too much as a solution, and its complementarity to other routes forgotten. Nonetheless, boundaries are being pushed back and times may well be about to change.

The readers of this book should therefore be aware that it has been written not as a 'cookbook' of recipes describing all the available methods for evaluating biocompatibility, past or present. Such literature can be found in profusion elsewhere, and it would be pointless to repeat the large amount of technical details available. It is not another revised edition either, but in fact a completely different perspective upon the problems and challenges in this field which need to be understood and put firmly into context. It reflects the requirements of, and the part that a more 'horizontal' approach has to play in, the evaluation of biocompatibility through international expert viewpoints on appropriate current and future developments. It has been designed specifically to address the general lack of knowledge relating to:

- the rapid development of regulations and standards over recent years in the biomedical field
- the principles behind the correct interpretation and use of such regulations and standards
- the test methods necessary as part of the evaluation of safety of medical materials and devices
- the current problems and needs/requirements of biomaterials
- the importance of issues relating to standardisation and quality of testing
- the forthcoming role that risk analysis will play in evaluating biological safety.

The book commences with a chapter on the current status of the implementation and interrelation of both sets of European and international standards on the biological evaluation of medical and dental materials and devices. Experts from both sides of the Atlantic consider the structure of standardisation relating to medical devices and the function of the standards within the framework of the European and US legislation, and the moves towards global harmonisation. The potential for revision and extension of the standards in the future is considered from each viewpoint and ties in with the subsequent chapters as appropriate.

The book continues to set the scene with four chapters which consider materials-related issues pertaining to the problems and needs/requirements of biomaterials. For the reasons already stated, there is no detailed consideration of the different categories of materials available for use as medical devices, nor is there discussion of the present and emerging applications for such materials. In the first of these chapters, aspects relating to the potential role of standardised test protocols/methodologies and CRMs and the application of internal quality control (QC) and external quality assessment (QA) measures are considered in detail. In the second, the major failure mechanisms relating to material (bio)degradation and the existing and proposed future test methods for assessing the production of degradation products and their effect on the body and the device (or material) properties are discussed. The current guidance on, and factors worthy of careful consideration in, toxicokinetic study design (absorption, distribution, metabolism and excretion of foreign compounds in the body with time) for degradation products and leachables are highlighted. The chapter ties in closely with the final chapter on the assessment of biological safety–risk analysis by considering the need to study risk assessment when evaluating degradation. The third chapter considers the concept of a 'dynamic' (polymeric) material surface, with the importance of, and yet the inherent difficulties associated with, available characterisation methodologies being discussed and views on appropriate future ways forward being presented. The last of these chapters outlines the current and future requirements for the validation and routine monitoring of sterilisation procedures, and associated allowable residue limits, for medical devices designed for patient contact.

The remaining five chapters examine the issues associated with the major general techniques for evaluating the important interactions of materials with their biological environment, and vice versa. They do not, however, consider either the effects of direct contact of implanted materials with living tissue or general animal welfare. Nor, therefore, do they consider potential sensitisation or irritation attributable to leachable endogenous or extraneous substances present in or on a medical device. These aspects have all been covered amply elsewhere in the literature. The first of these discusses the general principles behind the existing standard *in vitro* cell culture methodologies (including their inherent limitations) for assessing the toxic effect of device materials and/or extracts therefrom. Current moves relating to modification of the international standard, and the associated role a proposed collaborative trial has to play in this, are highlighted. The concept of apoptosis is also considered, there also being a close link with the later chapter discussing genotoxicity, carcinogenicity and reproductive toxicity.

The classification of categories of devices intended for use in contact with blood, and the rationale and current guidance for the structured selection of tests for evaluating blood interaction, together with the principles and the scientific basis for them, is presented in the second of these chapters. Device-specific issues in the structured selection of tests and future perspectives are also considered. The principles and methods for estimating the potential of medical materials and devices to induce genetic alteration or increase the incidence of neoplastic formation are discussed in the third chapter. The case for validated, standardised short-term tests which can be relied upon to predict long-term effects and clinical performance is also put forward. The link to the earlier cytotoxicity chapter on aspects of apoptosis should be noted. In the fourth chapter, the current perspectives, principles and future goals for an appropriate approach to morphological analysis of a range of explanted biomaterials as a means of providing guidance and assessment of efficacy and safety of such materials and devices are discussed. The final chapter of this section, and indeed the book, addresses the important emerging area of assessing the acceptability of risk and judging biological safety. Risk analysis is an essential part of this activity. Current thinking on the investigation of the safety of a medical device by identifying the hazards and estimating the risks associated with that device is presented. This chapter ties in with the earlier chapter which considered toxicological study design.

Through this approach it is believed that the book addresses the highlighted problems by providing:

- a complete account of the status of relevant standards and Directives
- an awareness of the principles and advice on their interpretation
- both a current and forward assessment of selected 'horizontal' test methodology by acknowledged experts in their field
- the issues associated with adopting the VAM approach, including validation of standardised methods, CRMs, and inter- and intralaboratory testing.

It is difficult to cover all aspects involved in such a complex and rapidly changing field, but the major considerations are presented here. These should allow the reader to gain an insight and/or a deeper appreciation of current efforts in this field and the future possibilities for improved biocompatibility evaluation. Where appropriate, this book can easily be supplemented by more detailed work in specific individual areas. It is now up to each and every reader, whatever their background and degree of experience (clinician, public or private sector scientist or administrator, regulator etc.), to actually implement their specific experience or general understanding, interests and capabilities within this framework of 'ideals' and to help take forward this field into a new era.

It should be noted that all the views expressed in the book are those of the respective authors and do not necessarily represent the policy of their affiliations.

I would finally like to express my appreciation to Sue Horwood, of Medi-Tech Publications, without whose initial drive and enthusiasm my thoughts and this book might never have been distilled into its present form. My thanks are also extended to all the contributors to the book, many of whom are now not just colleagues but also friends, and to everyone at Wiley for their cooperation during the publishing process.

Julian Braybrook
London, October 1996

# 1

# Biocompatibility Standards: An International Overview Part I: United States of America (USA)

DON MARLOWE

Office of Science and Technology, US Food and Drug Administration

## 1.1 INTRODUCTION

The evaluation of the biocompatibility of materials, i.e. the evaluation of the suitability of materials for use in implantable medical devices, has evolved over approximately the last 50 years. The first recognition of materials that did not cause an acute inflammatory response when placed in the human body concerned fragments of polymethylmethacrylate (PMMA) which splintered from the inner surface of the canopy of fighter planes during World War II. These splinters were often left to remain in place in tissues such as the eye because of the difficulty of removing them without causing further damage. However, only recently has the understanding of biocompatibility evolved to the point where some international agreement can be reached toward the systematic, biological evaluation of materials. This chapter outlines the current status of this discussion, focusing initially on the perspective from the USA and then from Europe.

## 1.2 HISTORICAL DEVELOPMENT OF BIOCOMPATIBILITY STANDARDS

In the USA, Autian (1961) was the first to describe a systematic approach to the evaluation of materials in the determination of their biological response. This scheme for testing was codified by the US Pharmacopoeia (USP) through its inclusion into the chapter concerning plastic containers (USP, 1965). This chapter described six classes for device plastics based on the response to a series of

*Biocompatibility Assessment of Medical Devices and Materials.*
Edited by Julian Braybrook. © 1997 John Wiley & Sons Ltd.

*in vivo* animal tests for which extracts, materials and routes of administration were clearly described. The Autian test scheme is still described in the current USP Monograph 88 concerning *in vivo* biological reactivity tests. It was not until well after 1976, when the medical device amendments to the Food, Drug and Cosmetic Act were passed, that the sixth class of the USP chapter was accepted as the norm for evaluating biocompatibility of materials used in medical devices and implants. This particular test method required the implantation of the material into rabbits for periods up to 120 hours and is still cited regularly as an indication of material biocompatibility.

When the medical device amendments were indeed established, the responsibility for the evaluation of devices, and the determination that they were safe and effective for their intended use, rested with the US Food and Drug Administration (FDA). This law clearly established that the FDA was responsible for regulating devices, not materials. This distinction is often not clearly understood or enunciated: often a very fine line must be drawn between a device and the material from which it is produced. However, any reflection on a material which is to be used in several types of devices shows that the material might be safe in contact with one type of tissue but very toxic on contact with another type. As a result, there was a need to broaden the spectrum of the types of tests called for to establish biocompatibility beyond the concepts in USP Monograph 88. The type of tissue, duration of implantation and relevant reactive end-point in the tissue had also to be considered.

Some 6 years later, the American Society for Testing and Materials (ASTM) published its standard (ASTM, 1982) which was developed over a period of several years by the ASTM Committee F04 on medical and surgical devices and materials. This document was the first to make use of a multiple variable or matrix scheme suggested by Autian's work: a manufacturer need only refer to the matrix, determine the type of tissue contacted and the duration of implantation. The scheme directed the manufacturer to consider only those types of tests judged to be actually necessary. Committee F04 also began the development of specific standardised testing protocols to be used in this work. Effort continues in these development areas today, including refinement of the F748 standard and development of new and revised testing protocols.

In 1987, the USA, United Kingdom (UK) and Canada published a guidance document in which the three countries agreed to 'harmonise' the process of evaluating biocompatibility through the determination of the tests required to show material biocompatibility in medical device marketing applications. The agreement utilised a matrix approach, similar to that used in the earlier ASTM F748 document and similar documents developed in both the UK (BS, 1979) and Canada (CSA, 1984). The agreement did not, however, specify any of the test methods called out by the selection matrix and, although well intentioned, caused considerable angst in countries who were not party to the tripartite discussions: how were similar evaluations among other countries to be harmonised? Nonetheless, the FDA effectively adopted this agreement as policy by directing reviewers of

**Table 1.1**   Contents of ISO 10993: Biological evaluation of medical devices

| | |
|---|---|
| Part 1 | Guidance on selection of tests |
| Part 2 | Animal welfare requirements |
| Part 3 | Tests for genotoxicity, carcinogenicity and reproductive toxicity |
| Part 4 | Selection of tests for interaction with blood |
| Part 5 | Tests for cytotoxicity: *in vitro* methods |
| Part 6 | Tests for local effects after implantation |
| Part 7 | Ethylene oxide sterilisation residues |
| Part 8 | Clinical investigation (not part of EN 30993) |
| Part 9 | Degradation of materials related to biological testing |
| Part 10 | Tests for irritation and sensitisation |
| Part 11 | Tests for systemic toxicity |
| Part 12 | Sample preparation and reference materials |

device applications to consider its recommendations as part of the device review process.

International discussions began in 1989 in the venue of a new, and currently operating, International Standards Organisation (ISO) Technical Committee (TC) 194 concerning biological evaluation of medical devices. ISO/TC 194 published the standard ISO 10993-1 (ISO, 1992) which also utilises a matrix approach as guidance. Other parts of ISO 10993 describe suggested test methods for evaluation of the several end-points of biocompatibility testing (Table 1.1), although the tests differ somewhat from both the earlier ASTM document and tripartite agreement.

Current review and revisions of both standards may serve to more closely harmonise their requirements. There are currently over 12 such tests described to various levels of specificity.

In 1995, the FDA Office of Device Evaluation (ODE) re-evaluated the policy of reviewing medical device applications using the tripartite agreement. Its Director issued new guidance (ISO, 1995) to the recommended biomaterials review process according to the requirements cited in ISO 10993-1. Allowances were, however, made for several variances with the international standard where established ODE policy in specific areas was in conflict with the standard. A copy of the matrix of tests to be considered is shown in Figure 1.1a, b and c.

## 1.3   FDA POLICY REGARDING USE OF STANDARDS FOR BIOCOMPATIBILITY TESTING

In 1980, the US Office of Management and Budget (OMB) published the directive, Circular A-119 (OMB, 1980), the express aim of which was to move the US government agencies away from the internal development of specifications and standards towards the use of similar documents developed in the voluntary consensus standards development sector. For example, under the mandate of A-119, the US Department of Defense and General Services Administration

| Device categories | | | Biological effect | | | | | | | |
|---|---|---|---|---|---|---|---|---|---|---|
| Body contact | | Contact duration<br>A- limited (≤24 h)<br>B- prolonged (24 h to 30 days)<br>C- permanent (>30 days) | Cytotoxicity | Sensitisation | Irritation or intracutaneous reactivity | Systemic toxicity (acute) | Subchronic toxicity (subacute toxicity) | Genotoxicity | Implantation | Haemocompatibility |
| Surface devices | Skin | A | X | X | X | | | | | |
| | | B | X | X | X | | | | | |
| | | C | X | X | X | | | | | |
| | Mucosal membrane | A | X | X | X | | | | | |
| | | B | X | X | X | O | O | | O | |
| | | C | X | X | X | O | X | X | O | |
| | Breached or compromised surfaces | A | X | X | X | O | | | | |
| | | B | X | X | X | O | O | | O | |
| | | C | X | X | X | O | X | X | O | |
| External communicating devices | Bloodstream, indirect | A | X | X | X | X | | | | X |
| | | B | X | X | X | X | O | | | X |
| | | C | X | X | O | X | X | X | O | X |
| | Tissue/bone/dentine communicating[1] | A | X | X | X | O | | | | |
| | | B | X | X | O | O | O | X | X | |
| | | C | X | X | O | O | O | X | X | |
| | Circulating blood | A | X | X | X | X | | O[2] | | X |
| | | B | X | X | X | X | O | X | O | X |
| | | C | X | X | X | X | X | X | O | X |
| Implant devices | Tissue/bone | A | X | X | X | O | | | | |
| | | B | X | X | O | O | O | X | X | |
| | | C | X | X | O | O | O | X | X | |
| | Blood | A | X | X | X | X | | | X | X |
| | | B | X | X | X | X | O | X | X | X |
| | | C | X | X | X | X | X | X | X | X |

**Figure 1.1**   General programme memorandum - #G95-1
A: Initial evaluation tests for consideration*
x is ISO evaluation tests for consideration
o is additional tests which may be applicable
[1] tissue includes tissue fluids and subcutaneous spaces
[2] for all devices used in extracorporeal circuits.
* see **B** for supplementary evaluation tests.

| Device categories | | | Biological effect | | | |
|---|---|---|---|---|---|---|
| Body contact | | Contact duration<br>A-limited ($\leq$24 h)<br>B-prolonged (24 h to 30 days)<br>C-permanent (>30 days) | Chronic toxicity | Carcinogenicity | Reproductive/Developmental | Biodegradation |
| Surface devices | Skin | A | | | | |
| | | B | | | | |
| | | C | | | | |
| | Mucosal membrane | A | | | | |
| | | B | | | | |
| | | C | O | | | |
| | Breached or compromised surfaces | A | | | | |
| | | B | | | | |
| | | C | O | | | |
| External communicating devices | Blood path, indirect | A | | | | |
| | | B | | | | |
| | | C | X | X | | |
| | Tissue/bone/dentine communicating | A | | | | |
| | | B | | | | |
| | | C | O | X | | |
| | Circulating blood | A | | | | |
| | | B | | | | |
| | | C | X | X | | |
| Implant devices | Tissue/bone | A | | | | |
| | | B | | | | |
| | | C | X | X | | |
| | Blood | A | | | | |
| | | B | | | | |
| | | C | X | X | | |

**Figure 1.1** (*continued*)
B: Supplementary tests for consideration
x is ISO evaluation tests for consideration
o is additional tests which may be applicable.

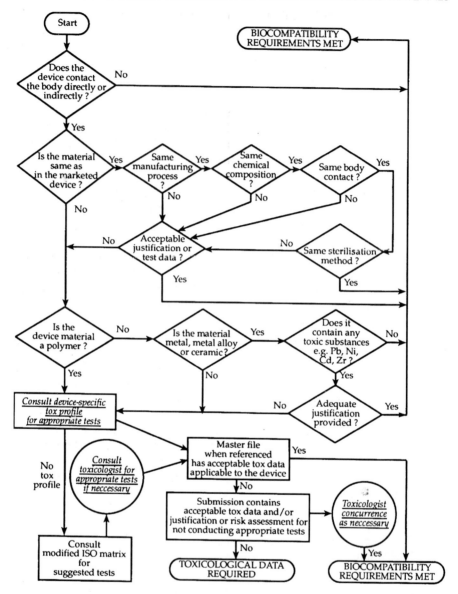

**Figure 1.1**   (*continued*)
**C:** Biocompatibility flowchart for the selection of toxicity tests for 510(k)s

ceased the development of specifications for the purchase of otherwise commercially available products in favour of specifications developed by organisations such as the ASTM and the Automotive Engineers. This OMB policy was reaffirmed in 1982 and 1993 with added emphasis on the use, where appropriate, of international standards. The FDA has also slowly increased the utilisation of consensus standards in the management of the risks related to medical devices. The FDA first published a policy related to the use of consensus standards for Class II (medium risk) medical devices (FDA, 1980) and this has been revised and strengthened in a succession of statements (FDA, 1981, 1985; CDRH, 1993). Recently, it published a general policy related to such standards for use across all sections of the Agency (FDA, 1995). In the area of biocompatibility, however, the FDA was reluctant to immediately embrace the suggested testing schemes described in the various national and international consensus documents. As the tripartite biocompatibility agreement was in place, the FDA perceived that there was some advantage to waiting until more experience had been gained with ISO 10993. The recent revision to clarify some points has led to the change in the 'Blue book' policy memorandum, as noted above. However, the FDA feels that the current provisions of ISO 10993 are not yet complete: several practices described in ISO 10993 do not agree with current US practice. Currently, most of the recommended ISO 10993 test method Parts describe several possible tests rather than a specific test, and this failure is seen as an area for considerable future development. Hence, the 'Blue book' memorandum suggests several additional tests which manufacturers are asked to consider in the evaluation of their devices.

This last point brings into focus the difficulties that must be overcome in the development of a globally harmonised set of biocompatibility requirements. Yet it should be noted that, as stated by the Director of the FDA Centre for Devices and Radiological Health (CDRH) at the meeting of the task force on international global harmonization in June 1995, the FDA is firmly committed to the concept. His comments outlined a measured approach to implementation of a harmonised set of requirements. Standards such as ISO 10993 are one of the foundations of global harmonisation.


## 1.4 FUTURE DEVELOPMENTS FOR BIOCOMPATIBILITY TESTING

During the process of revision of ISO 10993 to address a number of editorial difficulties noted since its first approval, several additional sets of comments were received. Their discussion may suggest a direction for a further revision of the standard, e.g. consideration of the differences between the matrices of the standard and those of the FDA 'Blue book', although other equally valid points are to be considered.

Hence it has been suggested that, for ISO 10993 to reach its maximum usefulness, the standard should describe the method(s) by which each type of suggested test is executed and the measures of their acceptable performance. Such test methods should be very specific regarding protocols and should be validated through international interlaboratory comparison trials. Estimates of the inter- and intralaboratory variations (and uncertainty) for such methods should be established. In this way, data derived from such testing can be compared between investigators and compared to existing information about the behaviour of materials in specific exposure environments. This should lead to the development of databases of material biological performance much like the physical property databases which now exist for many materials. Recent discussions in ISO/TC I94 Working Group (WG) 5 related to the development of a standard protocol and certified reference materials, CRMs, for *in vitro* cytotoxicity testing point the way forward. The availability of such standardised test methods is a necessary step in the global harmonisation process. This concept of valid analytical measurement (VAM) is therefore discussed more fully in Chapter 2 and again, more specifically to cytotoxicity, in Chapter 6.

Finally, recent discussions of a new approach to biocompatibility testing, based on knowledge of the chemical constituents of a material and the use of existing knowledge of the toxicity of the identified chemical constituents, holds the promise of limiting the amount of device-specific materials toxicity testing that might be required to support a medical device application. Such a concept requires the use of a standard unique identifier nomenclature for the constituents that go into the formulation of a material, and the knowledge base to link the material identifiers to the toxicity data. The FDA and US industry are actively discussing the development of these systems.

## 1.5   CONCLUSIONS

Biocompatibility testing in the USA has been evolving rapidly over the last 30 years. The standards which have been developed to codify the developments in this area are still not universally accepted in the global community, but considerable work has been identified for the future development of specific testing protocols, the re-evaluation of the underlying requirements for biocompatibility testing and, in the more distant future, new concepts for making more relevant decisions at lower cost to manufacturers and evaluators.

# Part II: Europe

MARJA KUIJPERS AND JAN-WILLEM DORPEMA
Laboratory for Medicines and Medical Devices, Rijksinstituut voor
Volksgezondheid en Milieu

## 1.6  INTRODUCTION

The need for the development of European standards (ENs) within the field of
medical devices arose from the new, harmonised legislative system based on the
so-called 'new approach' policy, introduced by the then European Economic
Community (now the European Union, EU) for this class of products (EC, 1994).
This legislation has to date been laid down in the two Directives regarding
medical devices, the Directive on Active Implantable Medical Devices (90/385/EEC)
(EC, 1990) and the Directive on Medical Devices (93/42/EEC) (EC, 1993).

Based on this policy, European legislation is restricted to basic safety
requirements, the task of detailed harmonisation being transferred to European
standardisation. A Directive can be considered to be a piece of Community
legislation. Once adopted, the Member States are obliged to transpose the
Directive into national law, thereby leading to 'harmonisation' of legislation and
the removal of technical barriers to trade. It should be noted that the provisions
of the Directives do not automatically become effective in Member States, certain
preliminary steps needing to be taken. To enable their implementation, each
Directive specifies dates by which Member States must execute the following steps:

- adopt and publish laws, regulations and administrative provisions necessary to
  allow implementation. Member States may adapt existing regulatory structures
  and do not need to use identical approaches, although the national laws and
  regulations must refer to the relevant Directive
- actual implementation of the Directives. This is the date from which manufacturers
  can begin to use the provisions/requirements
- accept products placed on the market based on compliance with national
  requirements, where they exist, for a transitional period, after which all
  products covered by a particular Directive should carry the equivalent CE mark.

Eventually, however, the Directives will replace any existing national systems
on product safety and performance in each Member State, although it should
be noted that the Directives include a derogation clause in the conformity
assessment procedures allowing national Competent Authorities to authorise,

within their individual countries, the marketing of individual products that have not complied with required conformity assessment procedures provided that 'the use is in the interest of protection of health'.

As indicated above, the Directives include 'essential requirements' (set out in the Annex belonging to them) which describe, in general terms, the safety aspects which have to be taken into account and met before the CE mark can be affixed and the product sold throughout the EU. These can be divided into two sections, the first dealing with general requirements, the second with requirements concerning design and construction. In paragraph 7 of this latter section, four main aspects of safety for medical devices are mentioned:

- chemical safety, related to the toxicological properties of the product and its components
- microbiological safety, related to the microbiological properties of the product
- physical safety, related to the physical properties of the material (e.g. mechanical, electrical, morphological), and the design and performance of the product
- biological safety, related to the biocompatibility of the product, which in fact comprises all chemical, physical and microbiological characteristics of the product and its component materials.

Hence 'the devices must be designed and manufactured in such a way as to guarantee the characteristics and performance referred to in the first section on general requirements. Particular attention must be paid to the compatibility between the materials used and biological tissues, cells and body fluids, taking account of the intended purpose of the device' (paragraph 7.1). Furthermore, 'particular attention must be paid to the tissues exposed and to the duration and frequency of exposure' (paragraph 7.2) and 'the device must be designed and manufactured in such a way as to reduce to a minimum the risks posed by substances leaking from the device' (paragraph 7.5).

Confirmation that these essential requirements have been met is achieved through one or more conformity assessment (certification) procedures. These procedures give manufacturers a choice of routes for CE mark authorisation of their products. In this phase the application of standards is indicated. The stringency of the procedures depends on which Directive applies and the classification of the product concerned. The classification system and the level of control applying are proportional to the degree of risk inherent in a medical device. The classification system consists of four classes: Class I (low risk), Classes IIa and IIb (medium risk) and Class III (high risk). For Classes IIa and IIb, and III, manufacturers must apply to a Notified Body (designated by a national Competent Authority) to carry out the conformity assessment procedure.

In summary, the following phases can be distinguished in the legislative procedure for the marketing of medical devices within the EU:

- classification of the product (in accordance with classification criteria laid down in the Directives on medical devices)

- selection and performance of the desired and appropriate conformity assessment
- affixation of the CE mark (in cases where conformity is declared, i.e. there is compliance with the essential requirements).

## 1.7 RELATIONSHIP BETWEEN STANDARDISATION AND LEGISLATION RELATING TO MEDICAL DEVICES

The relationship between European legislation and harmonised standardisation is that Directives require products to be safe and are mandatory, whereas standards are voluntary but offer the means to prove the safety. The basic requirement applying to a harmonised standard is that it must be fit to check for product compliance with the legislative safety requirements, i.e. the essential requirements.

Consequently, it was the European Committee for Standardisation (CEN) that was asked to develop, and put into effect, the necessary standards in order to enable and support implementation of the established medical device Directives, i.e. provide tools for the purpose of testing, certification and control of products. This has been achieved through the definition of the minimum levels of safety, quality, design and performance, and provision of recognised and validated test methods for product evaluation and comparison with defined specifications (CEN, 1995a).

However, within the field of medical devices, CEN also had to take measures to increase the efficiency in the development of ENs. One such step was the decision to define three different levels:

- Level 1: General standards (horizontal level)
  These are applicable to a broad range of products (all medical devices, all surgical implants) and deal with one or some aspects of safety. Horizontal standards, e.g. EN 30993 concerning biological evaluation of medical devices, are particularly suitable for laying down requirements and test methods regarding aspects inherent to many products.
- Level 2: Product group standards (semihorizontal level)
  These are applicable to a specific group of products and provide test methods as well as specifications for design, construction and use of materials.
- Level 3: Product (type) standards (vertical level)
  These are applicable to one or a few products and cover, in principle, all aspects of safety. A vertical standard may refer to a horizontal standard for general requirements or test methods, but can also provide specific additional requirements or indications for testing. It cannot, however, conflict with a horizontal standard, the latter governing the former.

In the process of developments of standards, preference is given to Level 1 standards, supplemented by Level 2 and Level 3 standards where necessary.

## 1.8   CEN ORGANISATION

Technical specifications ensuring compatibility between products, appropriate levels for their safety, quality or efficiency, and the test methods needed to establish conformity to these specifications have naturally tended to be set by national standards bodies. Although these may have developed in an equivalent manner, most notably within the framework of ISO, they may also vary from one country to another. Gradually, though, most national documents are being replaced by a single set of ENs forming a coherent technical background to the benefit of all. CEN is the organisation responsible for the planning, drafting and adoption of such standards through procedures which guarantee respect for transparency, consensus, national commitment and technical coherence. The CEN structure comprises a technical management system organised around the main sectors of CEN's activities (Sector Technical Boards), and standards drafting bodies as TCs and their WGs (CEN, 1993). CEN/TC 206 is the relevant committee concerning standards for biological evaluation of medical materials and devices.

Once the need for an EN has been established and it does not appear possible to use an existing reference document (or one under development, e.g. issued by ISO), a team of experts (originating from different research institutes, universities, industries etc.) is established as a TC. They do not represent professional/technical societies or trade associations, but the official members of CEN, i.e. the national standards bodies. CEN has 18 official members, of which 12 are standardisation institutes from EU Member States and six from EFTA countries. When consensus is reached on a draft standard in the TC, a procedure designed to ensure its general acceptability is then started. This includes a public enquiry and adoption of the standard through a formal vote by each national CEN member. ENs are ratified in the three official CEN languages, but formal adoption is only complete once the standard has been transposed into a national standard for each CEN member (CEN, 1994).

## 1.9   BIOLOGICAL EVALUATION OF MEDICAL DEVICES
(EN 30993, 1993–1996) (Kuijpers, 1995)

European activities concerning the standardisation of biological evaluation of materials commenced concurrently (in 1989) with the emerging activities within this field in the US. The scope of CEN/TC 206 was to consider the work of ISO/TC 194 and other relevant standardisation committees, in order to speed up the work of these TCs, harmonise European views of the field and ensure priority of projects mandated by the EC in connection with the medical device Directives. In other words, CEN/TC 206 was not requested to produce standards on its own but, in conformity with the CEN/ISO (Vienna) agreement on exchange of technical information, to accompany international developments within this field. Having said this, however, in case the European needs could not be met by application of these developments, CEN/TC 206 was to standardise test methods for biological evaluation for application by European countries. Thus a CEN/TC 206 working programme was drafted, specifically geared to the European situation. One of its main aims was to create practical tools to enable the implementation of the new European legislation on medical devices. The standards were to detail the safety requirements for the products included in this legislation and, by means of their application, enable the demonstration of conformity with the essential requirements. Discussions with ISO/TC 194 were organised to reach consensus on the content of both work programmes. Based on this consensus CEN/TC 206 decided to cooperate with ISO/TC 194 and to adopt the future standards produced by ISO/TC 194 as ENs.

Thus the development of the series of standards for biological evaluation of medical devices mainly took place within the organisational structure of ISO. Experts appointed by CEN Member States participated in the ISO WGs, but the decision-making process resulting in ENs took place by means of separate procedures within CEN. Initially, in the context of the harmonised technical legislation, the European Commission (EC) and European Free Trade Association (EFTA) only mandated the development of Level 1 standards. A number of important horizontal standards, e.g. quality systems for medical devices, methods and guidance on the valid routine control of sterilisation procedures, and clinical investigation of medical devices, were issued. Additionally, a standard was produced which considered the evaluation of biological safety and included all aspects of the biocompatibility of materials and medical devices; the biological safety is determined by the probability that inherent hazards (biological, chemical etc.) constitute real risk(s) during use of the medical device/product, and the nature and extent of those risks.

The new series of standards received the numbering EN 30993. To date, in addition to the general Part 1 regarding the testing of biological safety, a further 11 parts (which constitute the major part of the original working programme of CEN/TC 206) have been finalised and issued officially as ENs. As already mentioned (Section 1.8), these parts were based mainly on existing national standards and guidelines on biological testing of materials and devices. An additional important contribution was provided by the tripartite agreement, also discussed earlier. Within ISO they have also been published as the ISO series 10993. The series still is extending and five new parts are in preparation or being planned. Experience indicates that some of these various parts of the standard already need revision.

### 1.9.1 ISO 10993 (EN 30993) PART 1: GUIDANCE ON SELECTION OF TESTS

The most important part of the standard EN 30993 (equivalent to ISO 10993) is Part 1, which describes a standardised procedure to generate a systematic approach for the biological evaluation of every type of medical device. It specifies the minimal requirements for a proper evaluation of biological safety and the rationale behind the need for tests and their selection. It is not a 'one-way checklist' of tests; it does not prescribe whether, and which, specific tests have to be performed. A demonstrated history of use in a specified role equivalent to that of the device under design may result in the conclusion that no testing is required. The part also does not specify acceptance criteria per test or between tests. As such, therefore, it solely provides guidance and leaves the final decision up to the experienced practitioner (CEN, 1995b). The main items covered by Part 1 are:

• formulation of basic principles regarding biological evaluation within the framework of safety assessment.

   One of the major principles upon which the biological evaluation process is built is the concept of biological safety or biocompatibility. It used to be an acceptable concept that biocompatibility was equated with inertness and that the achievement of chemical stability was synonymous with achieving the goal of the universally biocompatible material. This no longer appears to be the case: the first consideration must be fitness for purpose (having regard for the characteristics and properties of the material). This concept leads to the second important point in the assessment of the biocompatibility of a material: a material should always be evaluated in its final state, so that it is in its end-use application and situation. The biocompatibility of a product is determined by various factors of diverging nature, e.g. material and surface characteristics, design, construction and manufacturing. Material and product characteristics included are the toxicological properties of the materials and their constituent components, the leaching and degradation potential of the materials (e.g. after ageing or temperature fluctuation), the resistance to heat (e.g. in the case of steam sterilisation, chemicals, UV or gamma irradiation) and the physical, mechanical and morphological properties (e.g. strength, melting point, surface properties, elasticity, porosity and conductivity). The physical characteristics of the final product (e.g. design, shape and performance) also contribute to biocompatibility. Finally, the microbiological properties of the product, e.g. whether it is sterile or not, also have an effect. In the final product, all these aspects are related and interact together. Thus, in essence, the biological safety of a medical device can be equated with its chemical, microbiological and physical safety. The nature, performance and interpretation of the test programme selected for biological evaluation of a device is of major importance. Several aspects should be taken into account, e.g. the chemical composition of the materials and their physical behaviour, the conditions of exposure of the device in the normal intended use (including the nature, degree, frequency and duration of contact), and the existing information available from literature, experience and tests.

• procedure for the identification and characterisation of the biological hazards potentially related to a product

   For the identification and characterisation of potential biological hazards related to the intended use, application and purpose of a specific medical device, its constituent materials and components, the processing steps leading to the final product, and the final product itself, must be identified and characterised. EN 30993 Part 1 provides several aspects to be taken into consideration when performing such an analysis.

• procedure for the evaluation of the real exposure, and assessment of the resulting effect, with regard to the biological hazards identified by means of selection and performance of appropriate tests

Following the identification of potential biological hazards, the risks constituted by them can be assessed by evaluation of the exposure on the one hand and, on the other, by evaluation of the biological effects exerted by them.

In summarising the content of EN 30993-1 the biological evaluation process must always start with the identification of the intended use and application of the device, followed by the characterisation and evaluation of the exposure of the device to the body. To facilitate this characterisation the standard has designed categories in terms of nature, duration and frequency of contact between the device and the human body. By categorising the device according to the indications in the standard, potential biological hazards to be considered can be identified. The standard gives guidance on which hazard should be considered for which type or category of device. Evaluation of the exposure to the potential biological hazards is then identified by means of biological response tests for each of the relevant potential hazards. The assessment procedure, as described in the standard, takes into account both the biological safety and performance of the device, and one could conclude that it supersedes the traditional toxicological test system, which is exposure directed. Experience gathered over the last 20 years, especially with the safety assessment of food and chemical substances, has shown the limitations of this approach; effect studies must be included to achieve rational predictive risk values.

## 1.9.2   REMAINING PARTS OF ISO 10993

The current, remaining parts of the standard (Parts 2–12 inclusive) are shown in Table 1.1. These specify tests for evaluating interactive behaviour between implant material and living tissue. This behaviour can be subdivided into two aspects, one concerning the host response and the other the material response. Five new parts of the standard are in development dealing with, among other things, test methods for the identification and quantification of degradation products from materials (Table 1.2).

## 1.9.3   PROBLEMS REMAINING TO BE ADDRESSED

Despite the development and availability of EN 30993, there are still situations where the application of the standard involves problems or shortcomings. Next

**Table 1.2**   New parts of EN 30993 currently in development

| | |
|---|---|
| Part 13 | Identification and quantification of degradation products from polymers |
| Part 14 | Identification and quantification of degradation products from ceramics |
| Part 15 | Identification and quantification of degradation products from coated and uncoated metals and alloys |
| Part 16 | Toxicokinetic study design for degradation products and leachables |
| Part 17 | Material characterisation |

to reasons of misunderstanding or misinterpretation, these situations mainly concern material-related aspects of biological safety and performance, not yet included in the standard. The aspects to which this applies are degradation of materials (followed by bioavailability of degradation products) and inflammatory and immunotoxic reactions to materials and degradation products. The standard does not yet include an appropriate strategy on how to trace or predict these kinds of problems; nor does it provide suitable test methods for the evaluation of these aspects. *In vitro* test methods, where the clinical situation can be simulated, are often not available and even animal tests sometimes cannot predict the interactions between the human body and the final product in its end-use application.

Another problem concerning application of the standard is the discrepancy between the test (*in vitro*) situation and end-use (*in vivo*) application. The relationship between the results obtained by each situation cannot always be linked unambiguously to each other. One of the reasons for this phenomenon is the higher sensitivity of *in vitro* tests compared to *in vivo* tests. However, even though *in vitro* cytotoxicity testing is therefore often used in the first, basic safety screen of materials, such testing may result in rejection of materials of use in specific applications where a small degree of cytotoxicity is acceptable. It is therefore very difficult to assess criteria for evaluation of *in vitro* test results, because in the end the assessment of safety must be based on end-use application and performance.

## 1.10   CONCLUSIONS

Despite the present availability of many standards, the evaluation of a medical device (in accordance with the essential requirements laid down in the European legislation) is a complex procedure. The Directives require a medical device to be assessed based on its safety and effectiveness/performance in its human application. As a consequence, the evaluation of a medical device is comprised of several different aspects. A considerable number of standards have already been generated, varying from horizontal Standards which cover general safety and performance aspects of the product assessment procedure to vertical product group or product-type Standards specifying product characteristics. However, the final safety and performance assessment of a medical device refelcts a complex process. Results of tests of different natures (dealing with chemical, biological as well as physical safety) have to be combined with results from clinical studies to produce an overall evaluation. Recognising the complexity of these evaluations, experts have been very reluctant to introduce acceptance criteria in the standards. However, the absence of such criteria has necessitated an additional standardised assessment system. For this reason general applicable standards regarding the qualification of systems and organisations, have been developed. Moreover, as the medical devices Directive intends to prevent an uncontrollable growth of test- and product-specific standards and the resulting overtesting, the development of qualification standards should be promoted to counterbalance this tendency.

Horizontal standards (which exclusively cover the pre-market compartment of the product lifecycle, taking into account the intended use) cover a large number of products with different intended purposes, but as a result they specify no, or few, acceptance criteria. For this reason some uncertainty in the evaluation will remain. This uncertainty must be evaluated by means of risk analysis.

Experiences related to the post-market compartment demonstrate that the (standard-based) conformity data and subsequent assessment by Notified Bodies cannot consistently guarantee the products to be safe and performing well, i.e. they do not efficiently predict effectiveness.

Based on the experience gained to date in the application of EN 30993, for the assessment of biological safety of a device during its intended use and application, there is a need for more specific test methods focused on end-use application and performance criteria. The end-use application is very important, but not always known in advance. For that reason the approach to biological evaluation and study design for a particular device is of major importance with regard to the reliability of the outcome. The biological evaluation procedure should consider *in vitro* and, if necessary, *in vivo* tests. It must be concluded with a clinical evaluation of the biological safety and performance. Part 1 of the standard should always be the basis of the biological evaluation strategy. For the specific implementation and performance of the test programme other parts of the standard, and semihorizontal and vertical standards (Levels 2 and 3) can be employed. The latter, however, must always comply with the horizontal standard on the biological evaluation of medical devices.

It should also be noted that the basic strategy laid down in Part 1 of the standard requires the combination of both reductional and conceptual thinking. The problem emerging from this choice is the so-called 'procedural rationality', i.e. it questions how to value, relate, prioritise and balance the test results of different origins. The safety aspects included in the evaluation process cover a wide range, from exposure on a molecular level to whole-body performance assessment supplied by clinical evaluation. Its uniqueness lies in that it intends to integrate test results obtained from both reductional and conceptual-directed methods. Recognising that the procedures for the assessment of product safety and performance are complex, and that consequently the interpretation of the results allows a certain degree of freedom, testing introduces a degree of uncertainty. This uncertainty can be compensated for by the determination of the acceptable level of risk. The introduction of risk analysis complements the biological test and, moreover, functions as a mechanism to prevent overtesting. CEN has developed a draft standard specifically dealing with medical devices/risk analysis (prEN1441, 1994). Aspects important to this concept are discussed in further detail in the final chapter of this book.

Measures which can be applied to control uncertainty in the testing and evaluation of medical devices can be focused on two aspects:

* development of test acceptance criteria
  Uncertainty can be minimised through explicit and precise definition of acceptance criteria. Chemical and physical testing allows the exact determination of test limits and the degree of uncertainty substantiated. Once this has been achieved, tests can be validated. However, with regard to the general safety aspects of products, i.e. the biological safety of medical devices, it is impossible to define acceptance criteria applying to all groups and types of products. This has stimulated the development of test- and/or product-specific standards (Level 3). Consequently, the production of standards in the field of medical devices has shown an autonomous, uncontrollable growth. Historical experience in Europe indicates that this is a counterproductive phenomenon, creating bureaucracy and a subsequent decrease of mutual recognition. Subsequently, there is a need for supplementary mechanisms. It is also worth noting that in food and chemical control and safety assessment, where product performance is not involved, the traditional approach of defining and applying acceptance criteria did not prove to be a suitable predictor of risk/benefit balance for humans. To overcome this problem and to improve the assessment procedure, risk analysis has been introduced.

* qualification of systems, organisations and persons
  In addition to the introduction of risk analysis, the degree of uncertainty can be controlled by qualification of systems, organisations or persons involved in the testing and evaluation of medical devices. The baseline guarantee for the control of uncertainty is the implementation of, and accreditation to, a quality system. For laboratories it should preferably be based on the standard *General criteria for the operation of testing laboratories* (EN 45001, 1989), which represents the minimal quality infrastructure on top of which the performance of quality can be demonstrated. It is further intended that to demonstrate consistent quality and, concurrently, control and minimise the uncertainty, organisations shall qualify through performance evaluation schemes (yet to be established). Material certification studies (MCS) need to be carried out to establish benchmark values for components or properties of materials and CRMs for use in biological tests. The combination of a CRM with an appropriate standardised test methodology will also enable the exchange, recognition and comparison of test results produced in different places. This whole concept of valid analytical measurement is discussed in further detail in the next chapter.

## 1.11 REFERENCES

ASTM (1982) F748: standard practice for selecting generic biological test methods for materials and devices. ASTM, Philadelphia PA, USA.

Autian J (1961) Plastics: uses and problems in pharmacy and medicine. Am J Hosp Pharm 18:329–349.

BS (1979) BS 5736 Evaluation of medical devices for biological hazards, Part 1: Guide for the selection of biological methods of test. BSI, Milton Keynes, UK.

CDRH (1993) Policy on consensus standards: participation and use. Director's 'Blue book' policy memo. CDRH, Rockville MD, USA.

CEN (1993) Guidelines for technical committees. CEN, Brussels, Belgium.

CEN/CENELEC (1994) Internal regulations, Part 2: Common rules for standards work (edn. 1994-03). CEN, Brussels, Belgium.

CEN (1995a) Annual report 1994. CEN, Brussels, Belgium.

CEN (1995b) CEN memento 1995/1996. CEN, Brussels, Belgium.

CSA (1984) CAN3-Z310.6-M84: Testing for biocompatibility. Canadian standards Association (CSA), Toronto, Ontario, Canada.

EC (1990) Approximation of the laws of the Member States relating to active implantable medical devices (90/385/EEC). OJ L189 (20 July):17-24, EC, Brussels, Belgium.

EC (1993) Medical devices Directive (93/42/EEC). OJ L169 (12July):1-43, EC, Brussels, Belgium.

EC (1994) Guide to the implementation of Community harmonisation Directives based on the new approach and global approach, First version. Office for official publications of the EC, Luxembourg.

EN45001 (1989) General criteria for the operation of testing laboratories. CEN, Brussels, Belgium.

EN30993 Parts 1–12 (1993–1996) Biological evaluation of medical devices. CEN, Brussels, Belgium.

prEN1441 (1994) Draft standard on medical devices – risk analysis. CEN, Brussels, Belgium.

FDA (1980) Policy on Class II medical devices: 45. US Federal Register, FDA, Rockville MD, USA.

FDA (1981) Policy on Class II medical devices: 47. US Federal Register, FDA, Rockville MD, USA.

FDA (1985) Policy on Class II medical devices: 50(205). US Federal Register, FDA, Rockville MD, USA.

FDA (1995) International harmonisation, Policy on standards: 60(196). US federal register, FDA, Rockville MD, USA.

ISO (1992) Biological evaluation of materials Part 1: Selection of tests. ISO, Geneva, Switzerland.

ISO (1995) Use of international standard ISO 10993, Biological evaluation of medical devices Part 1: Evaluation and testing. Memo from ODE Director to reviewing staff, FDA, Rockville MD, USA.

Kuijpers MR (1995). Biocompatibility, development and application of standards. Collected papers of the 9th Intl. Conf. on Medical Plastics (ed. Skov HR), Amsterdam, The Netherlands.

OMB (1980) Circular A-119: Federal participation in the development and use of voluntary standards. US Office of Management and Budget (OMB), FDA, Rockville MD, USA.

USP (1965) The Pharmacopoeia of the USA, 17th revision: 902.

# 2

# The Role of Material Standardisation and Method Validation in Evaluating Biocompatibility

JULIAN BRAYBROOK
Laboratory of the Government Chemist, Teddington, Middlesex, UK

## 2.1 INTRODUCTION

Numerous analyses are performed worldwide every year for many reasons, on the basis of which many important decisions are taken. The accuracy of the data obtained is therefore a prerequisite for the correct interpretation of results and guaranteed assurance that the most appropriate decisions are reached. It also allows for the comparison of results, and yet it is this latter aspect especially which is often disregarded, with resulting economic consequences. For example, it has been reported previously that, in the United States, 10% of all clinical analyses required repeat testing at a cost of about $900 million (Cali, 1975). In Germany too, losses through poor performance by analytical laboratories have been estimated in the past to be about DM1 billion (Griepink, 1984).

Establishing such desired accuracy of analytical data through the assessment and demonstration of quality is therefore a major issue for society today. In the European Union (EU), all the policies connected with the completion of the internal market stress the importance of European standardisation contributing to the creation of a genuine competitive single market in which barriers to free movement of goods between Member States are removed. As indicated in the previous chapter, the 'new approach' technical harmonisation and 'global approach' evaluation of conformity has already made it possible to define a working framework in which European regulation can make use of the genuine harmonised method standards being developed. However, 'successful standardisation implies successful implementation. Credible certification, inspection and test procedures play a key role in creating the conditions which allow confidence

*Biocompatibility Assessment of Medical Devices and Materials.*
Edited by Julian Braybrook. © 1997 John Wiley & Sons Ltd.

to grow and mutual recognition of each Member State's procedures to become effective' (EC, 1990). As a result, a number of hurdles still need to be overcome.

In this context, analytical quality assurance (AQA) is assuming increasing importance. The majority of the principles of AQA are considered in some depth in the first part of this chapter as an indicative solution to the problem. These are then examined further in relation to the specific difficulties currently being experienced in the biomedical field.

## 2.2    THE PRINCIPLES OF AQA

It is acknowledged (Garfield, 1991; Parkany, 1993) that the more important features of an AQA programme include:

- the use of validated methodology
- properly maintained and calibrated equipment
- the use of (C)RMs
- effective internal quality control (QC) measures, e.g. statistical control principles (control charts)
- participation in interlaboratory tests (proficiency testing (PT) schemes)
- external quality assessment (QA) system by accreditation or other compliance schemes
- staff education and training
- a supporting infrastructure.

### 2.2.1   MEASUREMENT VALIDATION

The results of analytical measurements need to be fit for purpose, and the results obtained in different locations or at different times should be consistent. Valid measurements and agreement between laboratories can be achieved by adhering to basic principles compatible with modern quality systems (Sargent and MacKay, 1995).

The following are recognised as being the key acceptance criteria for the adoption of validated methodology:

- the methodology has been adequately studied, i.e. validated
- the method has met the required standard, i.e. through the use of statistical analysis
- the text of the methodology has been drafted in the correct format for the relative standards body.

#### 2.2.1.1   Performance Characteristics

Analytical measurements should be made to satisfy an agreed requirement, i.e. there should be a specific purpose, and only when this has been formulated can other crucial aspects be considered. These measurements should also be made

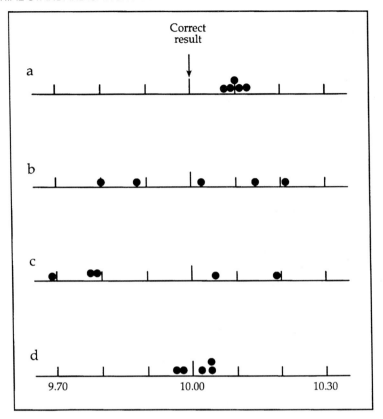

**Figure 2.1** Schematic showing precision and accuracy (reproducibility and repeatability). (a) Results precise but inaccurate; (b, c) Results imprecise but accurate; (d) Results precise and accurate

using methods which have been tested to ensure fitness for purpose, i.e. the measurement method needs to be tested against its specification to provide evidence that the performance characteristics will indeed be adequate for the intended use. The type and amount of effort required to validate a given method depends on both the former history of the method and the level of effort justified by the proposed application. Resulting limitations of the data must be clearly stated. The two most common factors relevant to achieving fitness for purpose relate to the requirement for data to provide relevant information and to the consequences which may arise as a result of errors in individual measurements. The performance characteristics that can be checked include selectivity, range, linearity, limit of detection, limit of determination, bias, precision,[1]

---

[1] A measurement process is sufficiently precise if it produces results for a RM which are statistically as precise as the precision of the measurement process participating in the certification programme, i.e. it is the closeness of agreement between two independent test results in a series obtained under prescribed conditions

repeatability,[2] reproducibility[3] and robustness (Figure 2.1). Collaborative testing enhances the confidence in the method and values obtained.

### 2.2.1.2    Precision and Bias

The precision of the whole method must be established, not simply that of the end determination. Any bias, i.e. systematic error, can be checked by the use of certified reference materials (CRMs) or, if these are unavailable, by comparison with another validated technique based as far as possible on different principles.

### 2.2.1.3    Uncertainty

All analyses are subject to an overall degree of uncertainty (Eurachem, 1994) and its sources should be identified and evaluated, regardless of the purpose of the results 'where it is relevant to the validity or application of the test result, where a client's instructions so require or where uncertainty affects compliance to a specification or limit'. It conveys the incompleteness of knowledge of the value being estimated by the measurement and, generally, comprises several components. Some of these can be evaluated from the statistical distribution of the results of a series of measurements. The remaining components are derived from alternative sources, e.g. instrument specifications, collaborative studies etc. Specific examples of where uncertainty can arise in analysis include operator bias, instrumental bias measurement condition, cross-contamination, computer software, reagent purity and sample effects.

### 2.2.2    CERTIFIED REFERENCE MATERIALS

Valid analytical measurements depend critically on the use of reliable standard materials, or RMs,[4,5] because it is through this mechanism that traceability[6] and hence comparability can be obtained, i.e. analytical measurements made in one location can be compared directly with those made elsewhere. In some sectors the use of appropriate, well-characterised RMs or calibration standards (which provide an external reference point and prevent loss of reliability of results caused by drifting with time) may be mandatory or possibly enforced by regulatory

---

[2] Repeatability describes the extent to which the same result can be obtained again and again using the same apparatus (when obtained by one operator), i.e. within-laboratory standard deviation

[3] Reproducibility describes the extent to which results are always the same, within experimental error, using different sets of apparatus (when obtained by different operators), i.e. between-laboratory standard deviation. It is the value below which the absolute difference between two single test results obtained with the same method on the identical test material under different conditions may be expected to lie within 95% probability [Mandel, 1971] [ISO, 1991]

[4] A RM is a material or substance for which one or more values are established sufficiently well to validate a measurement system [ISO, 1992]

[5] A CRM is a RM for which one or more property values are certified by a technically valid procedure accompanied by, or traceable to, a certificate or other documentation which is issued and certified by an organisation recognised as competent to do so [ISO, 1992]

[6] Traceability is the property or result of a measurement [ISO, 1984] whereby it can be related to appropriate standards, usually national or international, through an unbroken chain of comparisons

requirements. In others the benefits (and reasons) for usage may be less obvious and adoption may need to be encouraged.

The literature is replete with detailed reviews of specific RM categories and it is not the intention to repeat them here (ISO, 1982; Gladney *et al.*, 1987; Boumans and Roelandts, 1989; Roelandts, 1989). Instead, attention will be restricted to the more fundamental aspects and characteristics relevant to all RMs prior to discussion of the current and future issues pertaining to their potential relevance and use in the biomedical sector; there remains much confusion as to the 'uncertainties' attached to the values of elements in 'biological' RMs (Parr *et al.*, 1987).

RMs were first produced by the National Institute of Standards and Technology (NIST), formerly the National Bureau of Standards (NBS), in the USA at the beginning of the century, and shortly afterwards in Germany and the UK. However, it was the rapid evolution of analytical instrumentation in the 1950s that significantly increased the importance and usefulness of RMs. This necessitated the formation of an ISO RM Committee (ISO-REMCO), which establishes international guidelines on the principles of certification, methods of use, needs, and availability and nomenclature of RMs (ISO, 1981, 1989, 1992).

### 2.2.2.1 Types of RM

There are three types of RM:

- A single-substance CRM, e.g. pure solution/material (method standard), is an RM certified for chemical purity or some specific physical property. In the latter case (when produced according to recognised certification (ISO, 1989) and quality systems (ISO, 1995)), they act as transfer standards providing traceability of routine data to high-quality and well-documented primary standards.[7] Where the certified values have been determined using a definitive (absolute) measurement technique, the technically true value can be regarded as traceable to the base units of the SI system or their derivatives (Marchandise, 1987). Through the use of SI base units as true values, a measurement tree or pyramid has been established for transferring accuracy[8] throughout the measurement system via methods, transfer standards and RMs (Cali and Reed, 1976). However, it is difficult to relate these units to actual measurements of chemical composition as a result of matrix effects and the precision of analytical measurements being far more uncertain than the uncertainties related to measurement of the SI units. There is also the difficulty associated with the direct and unambiguous measurement of purity (Head, 1989), it only being possible to determine impurities by as many methods as possible.

---

[7] Primary standards are chemical standards designed or widely acknowledged to have the highest metrological qualities and whose values are accepted without reference to other standards.

[8] A measurement process is sufficiently accurate if it is precise and produces results for a RM which do not differ from the certified value by more than can be accounted for by within- and between-laboratory statistical fluctuations, i.e. it is estimated by proper evaluation of both systematic and random errors, and is the closeness of agreement between a test result and the accepted reference value

- A matrix CRM, e.g. pesticides in soil, is an RM whose matrix is the same as, or similar to, that of the material under analysis (with one or more of the analytes in the matrix certified).
- A method-dependent CRM, e.g. pure extract or solution (for testing the separation step), raw extract (for testing clean-up) or spiked sample (for assessing extraction recovery), is an RM employed for testing part(s) of an analytical procedure.

### 2.2.2.2  Uses of RMs

Prior to use, the suitability of the CRM should be confirmed with respect to certified value, precision, characterisation method, recommended sub-sample weight, and certification expiry date. An RM is suitable for use if its certified value for a selected characteristic of interest has a precision equal to or better than the average precision obtainable by analytical methods, either being used in its certification or considered for use in a particular application. It is desirable to have a measure of the quality of the certification data for the RM accounting for the degree of precision.

The most common use of RMs is as a monitor of a measurement system that is in a state of statistical control, i.e. a valid measurement procedure. As RMs are usually only available in small amounts, the statistics of the measurement process should be demonstrated by measurements on alternative materials. The results of an RM measurement can then be considered representative of that measurement system. The RM should be used on a regular basis, although sporadic usage upon observation of suspect data is also valid. CRMs may be employed as the sole RM or may be used with internal RMs produced in-house (through the application of CRMs).

Other uses of RMs include the establishment of measurement traceability (e.g. development of secondary RMs), evaluation and comparison of field methods, and to serve as method evaluators. It should be noted that measurement of a single RM may not be fully informative as it is impossible to indicate where any analytical errors involved actually lie.

### 2.2.2.3  RM Production

The rationale for producing RMs has been provided elsewhere in the form of a flow chart (Griepink, 1984). However, it is useful to expand on the more major points here. There are three main criteria, each of which can be further subdivided, for establishing RMs: selection, preparation and certification.

*Selection*

As already indicated, one of the first considerations should be the assessment of the technical requirements which will dictate the material's end use. This governs the certification requirements such as accuracy, stability and physical form of the material. It is also necessary to develop an adequate means of measuring the property values; preferably these are established on the basis of accuracy, i.e. the demonstrated relationship, or traceability, to the true property value. Often, though, such measurement is not possible; this is the situation where the relationship between some property and the parameter being measured cannot be established from a sound theoretical basis that can be expressed in mathematical terms. In such cases measurement comparability (i.e. measurements agreeing within the limits of uncertainty which reflect the end-use requirements (Cali, 1975; Coleman, 1980)) is best achieved through the use of arbitrarily selected RMs from a single source based on highly standardised methods of analysis and/or tests.

Furthermore, ideally the RM should have a similar (matrix) composition as the sample to be analysed, which it should also match with respect to levels and speciation (i.e. valency, and potential interference and binding patterns) of elements present (Taylor, 1983). In this way, as far as is possible, the same sources of error are encountered. Nonetheless, as a result of inherent error in the process, including that in the characterisation of the RM itself, the result produced by the measurement process is unlikely to be the same as the certified value. Acceptable limits for both precision and bias are therefore necessary to judge realistically the merit of the process in question (partly dependent on the mode of certification). The measurement process must produce results with accuracy (precision and trueness) within a tolerable bias.

## Preparation

During the preparation phase the following characteristics need to be addressed:

- A sufficient, long-lasting material stock should be available.
- Homogeneity with the minimum sample size should be verified (below this level the uncertainty caused by heterogeneity contributes around 30% of the uncertainty of the reference (or certified) values).
- Physical and chemical stability should be ensured over a suitable range of conditions appropriate to storage conditions or use.

Homogeneity with respect to the characteristic of interest is the most important property of an RM. Homogeneity testing is performed mostly on packaged, subdivided RM units assumed to be representative of the bulk. Heterogeneity is usually minimised by making the subsample size sufficiently large. Any differences are reflected in the uncertainty statement on the RM's accompanying certification document. Individual units are selected randomly and replicate analyses carried out on each of them, using a test portion size of the same magnitude as that employed by the average user's methods for the same characteristic, and a test method as precise as those methods. In a homogeneity study it is important that the techniques employed are highly precise; accuracy is less important.

The difference between representative measurements must be smaller than the overall uncertainty limits of the measurements (Marchandise and Colinet, 1983). This allows for heterogeneity of other characteristics, provided that they have no influence on the characteristic of interest. The balance between such factors means that assessment of a true value for a selected characteristic is theoretically impossible; the objective is therefore to yield an RM of sufficient trueness[9] for use in a reasonable number of common analytical applications.

Analysis of variance is one of the common statistical techniques employed to analyse the results. If the difference between the between-units variation and the within-unit variation is not statistically significant (ISO, 1990), the material is homogeneous. If there is a statistical significance, but the between-units variation is small from the user's point of view, then the material is sufficiently homogeneous. If the between-units variation is also significant, then the material is not homogeneous and should not be used as an RM.

The ideal RM should also be physically and chemically stable for an indefinite period of time. However, most materials undergo alteration under stimulus, so that changes in speciation, part(s) of the matrix or even the certified values may occur. Where stability is not infinite, an expiry date needs to be determined and provided on the RM's accompanying certification document.

### Certification

Certification is the process of obtaining property value data which approach as closely as possible to the true value, together with uncertainty limits. There are three procedures for achieving this (Marchandise, 1987):

- certification by a single laboratory
- certification based on statistical consensus of several laboratories
- certification based on several methods and several laboratories.

Depending on the type of RM, its end-use requirement, the qualification of the involved laboratories and the quality of the method or methods, one approach may be chosen as being most appropriate.

In certain circumstances certification can be carried out by a single laboratory using a definitive method (i.e. a method that is based on first principles, has a high precision and for which limits of uncertainty can be stated with high degree of confidence). Such methods frequently require specialised techniques, are often time-consuming and expensive, and usually require highly skilled personnel. There may also be an associated bias (e.g. owing to operator insufficiencies etc.) and a fair estimate of uncertainty may not be achieved. Furthermore, few definitive methods exist for organic analyses. Acceptance of such RMs requires user-community confidence. Hence, this procedure is generally used only where

---

[9] Trueness involves comparison between the mean of the laboratory measurement results and the certified value of the RM [Sutarno and Steger, 1985]

no alternative is available. A derivation of the procedure utilises a range (usually three) of reliable, independent (usually reference) methods of analysis for which both the accuracy and the precision are clearly known.

The second method consists of obtaining several laboratories' results and submitting them to statistical analysis (with rejection of individual values that appear to disagree with other values, i.e. outliers); the mean value is certified as the estimate of the true value. However, this approach should be treated with caution, as a large pool of results does not guarantee that the mean value will be the true value. Furthermore, the statistical treatment usually used may be unreliable.

Certified values are not expected to deviate from the true value by more than the stated measurement of uncertainty. Each laboratory mean is considered to be an unbiased estimate of the characteristic of interest. The mean of the laboratory means is assumed to be the best estimate of that characteristic. In such a programme, randomly selected units of the RM are distributed to participating laboratories, which each perform a predetermined determination from each unit, in replicate, for the characteristic of interest. The number of participating laboratories is determined by consideration of the precision of the estimates of standard deviations. It is most desirable to have 30 participating laboratories carrying out two determinations on one unit of RM. However, typically, 15 laboratories making three determinations suffices.

The third procedure is generally accepted to be the preferred method. When independent laboratories (often employing independent methods) produce results which are in agreement, bias can be assumed to be negligible and the overall mean value of the data set is accepted as the certified value and the best approximation of the true value. At least two or three experienced laboratories should participate for each method. Wherever possible definitive methods should be included in the procedure. Therefore, the uncertainty in the overall mean reflects the difference between the results reported by different laboratories and arises from the different methodologies selected and other laboratory-associated factors (e.g. environment, analyst and calibration etc.).

However, for complex CRMs, where many properties are to be certified, it is suggested that a combination of the above three procedures be employed, although it should be noted that just one method applied by only a few laboratories may be valid for certification purposes.

It is important to note that the analysis of interlaboratory data is an inferential process. For each set of data from participating laboratories, measures are inferred for the certified value of the characteristic of interest and its uncertainty. Complications can arise from data sets that do not meet the criteria for the valid application of a purely statistical approach, i.e. a normal distribution (with a minority of outliers) and a random (not systematic) error as the major cause of scatter. The decision on them is based on the available data and any background information on the data and process employed.

## 2.2.2.4  RM Certificate

Following statistical analysis, the data are distilled into one meaningful uncertainty statement for each value certified and included on the final certification document. An account needs to be taken of the precision of all the measurements and the homogeneity of the material, but it is the true value that is most important. ISO Guide 31 (ISO, 1981) clearly describes, in detail, the essential information to be included on certification documents, but this can be summarised as follows:

- the general particulars of the certifying organisation and the RM (name, sample, number, date of certificate etc.)
- a description of the material and its intended use
- the homogeneity limit (minimum size of representative sample)
- the certified value(s) of interest (i.e. the consensus value or mean of the laboratory means), the precision of this value (expressed as a confidence level or variance), the between-laboratory standard deviation (see Figure 2.2) and the within-laboratory standard deviation
- the material's expiry date
- references (e.g. accompanying reports indicating preparation and certification procedures, analytical data etc.) and the names of the participating analysts and certifying officers.

## 2.2.3  INTERNAL QUALITY CONTROL (QC)

QC can be defined as the mechanism (practical activities) established to control errors and forms a vital part of a comprehensive AQA programme (Thompson and Wood, 1995). All organisations carrying out analytical measurements should have well-defined QC activities.

Internal QC is generally accepted (IUPAC, 1993) as comprising the following three components:

- analytical performance characteristics, e.g. control charts etc.
- records, e.g. staff training and competence, equipment maintenance and calibration, and sample handling and disposal
- audit procedures.

Whatever analytical method is selected, its performance characteristics must be known in order to determine the uncertainty of bias attached to the results. The precision of the method should have been established by collaborative trial, but the repeatability of an individual laboratory may not be the same as that obtained in the interlaboratory trial, and reproducibility may not really be a property of the method as it represents bias (AMC, 1989). Day-to-day repeatability and assurance of controlled analysis in a laboratory can be monitored using control charts, with the availability of a sufficient amount of stable and

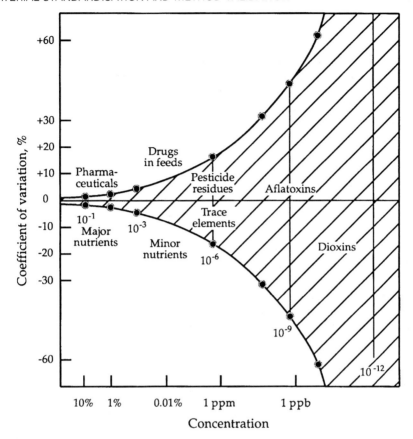

**Figure 2.2** Interlaboratory coefficient of variation as a function of concentration (reproduced with permission from Horwitz *et al.*, 1980)

homogeneous QC material for analysis with each batch of samples. Results are compared with the reference value. Control limits are established at three standard deviations above and below the reference value, and warning limits at two standard deviations. However, alternative plots are also possible, e.g. where small but consistent errors are detected. Nevertheless, control charts do not provide an indication of the overall trueness, or freedom from bias, unless the QC material is a CRM. When a laboratory uses a CRM to check its measurement process, the number of determinations should be at least 10. For a periodic check to ensure precision and/or trueness, duplicate determinations are sufficient, although the total number of replicates should be at least 10. More practically, however, the CRM is used simply to supplement the regular QC sample. Internal QC samples are commonly supplemented by external QC samples.

## 2.2.4  *EXTERNAL QUALITY ASSESSMENT (QA)*

QA, although frequently used interchangeably with QC, is actually the mechanism to verify that the system is operating within acceptable limits, i.e. the objective testing of the performance of a laboratory by an external agency. Its need arises because it is no longer sufficient just to obtain the correct answer: the accuracy or comparability of analytical data has to be demonstrable to all.

There are two main, essentially complementary, ways in which this can be achieved:

- PT schemes, where performance assessment is through interlaboratory comparisons of centrally distributed samples
- physical inspection, i.e. third-party (objective) assessment, or accreditation or other compliance scheme, to ensure that in-house QA procedures comply with established, recognised standards (within acceptable limits).

### 2.2.4.1  PT Schemes

PT schemes which comply with the internationally accepted protocol (Thompson and Wood, 1993) provide a regular, ongoing assessment of laboratory performance (see Figure 2.3) and are a more objective and independent assessment than that available through the use of CRMs.

Although there are many similarities between CRMs and PT schemes, differences also exist (Table 2.1) and so the two are only complementary and neither should be used to the exclusion of the other.

Such schemes are also cost-effective when sample throughput is high, as the samples can be incorporated easily into the work pattern; they are therefore frequently used as a convenient means of demonstrating quality for both internal purposes and/or customers and accreditation bodies.

There are two main types of PT scheme:

- for measuring laboratory competence in undertaking a very specific analysis, e.g. a specific element in a specific matrix
- for judging laboratory competence across a certain field or type of analysis, e.g. trace element analysis by a specific method.

Each type can be further subdivided into three categories:

- subsample distribution to participating laboratories (the most common type)
- successive sample circulation from laboratory to laboratory
- sample division, with each laboratory testing one part of each sample.

There are a number of clearly defined stages to the typical framework of a PT scheme:

- identification of the requirements of the proficiency test
- preparation and characterisation of the bulk material (usually by a single expert laboratory)

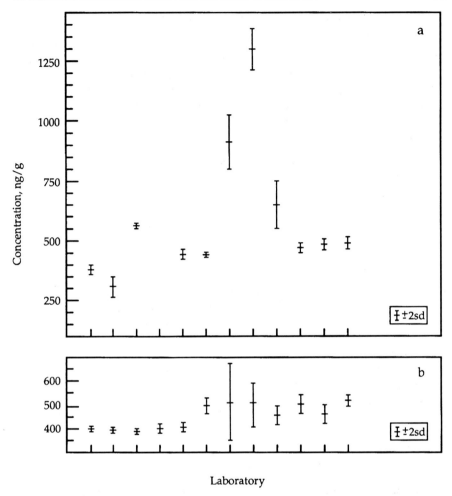

**Figure 2.3** Improvement in between-laboratory agreement for fish oil analysis. (a) 1990; (b) 1992

- (homogeneous) sample distribution to participating test laboratories (commonly four times per annum, so that laboratories are not discouraged from their own routine QC)
- sample analysis and data reporting by the test laboratories (commonly using their routine procedures)
- data evaluation and performance score assessment ('so-called' z-score[10])

---

[10] Z-score is calculated by taking the difference between the analyte value reported and the assigned value, then dividing by a target value for standard deviation [Horwitz, 1982]. A z-score of $<2$ is satisfactory, 2–3 is questionable and $>3$ is unsatisfactory. Alternatively, where there is no basis for a common value of standard error, q-scoring based on the relative bias, is sometimes used

**Table 2.1**  Comparison of the similarities and differences between CRMs and PT schemes

| CRMs | PT schemes |
|---|---|
| Assess/demonstrate the trueness of the data | Frequently assess data comparability rather than trueness (trueness only assessed if assigned value validated independently of participants' results) |
| Establish traceability of results to a recognised standard | Traceability is not normally provided |
| Must have a reasonable shelf-life | PT materials can be of shorter shelf-life (*ca.* one month) and so tend to be applied to less stable samples, e.g. blood |
| Certified values disclosed in advance to analyst | Assigned values are not disclosed until the test is completed, i.e. a more objective assessment |
| Certified values are established by procedures of known validity | Technical advice on methods etc. available from scheme organiser |
| Uncertainty of certified values is usually small | Assigned values often based on consensus of participants' results, which may be a biased estimate of the true value |
|  | Uncertainty of assigned values tend to be higher |

- notification of individual test laboratory performance scores
- commencement of the next round.

There are essentially three ways in which to determine a working estimate of the true value:
- addition of a known amount or concentration of analyte to an 'analyte-free' base material (a completely satisfactory method in many cases)
- use of a consensus value produced by a group of expert or referee laboratories using the best possible methods (closest approach to true value and indicative of accuracy, but often time-consuming and financially expensive)
- use of a consensus value produced in each round of a proficiency test, based on the results of the participants, i.e. the mean value following rejection of any outliers (the cheapest method, but difficult to obtain a real consensus and only indicative of comparability owing to the risk of producing a biased estimate of the true value, particularly where analysis is difficult. Furthermore, there is less frequent evaluation of the uncertainty of assigned values and thus traceability to a well-defined measurement method is not possible).

The standard deviation is selected as an estimate of the actual variation encountered in a particular round of the scheme, or a target value representing the maximum allowed variation consistent with achieving valid data. It often has to be derived when no other data on the variability of the target analysis are available (from collaborative trial or prescribed by legislation). Ancillary benefits, e.g. the opportunity to establish individual improvement(s), comparability of individual performance to peer laboratories at a particular time, and the relative merits of different analytical methodologies, can also be derived.

However, although PT schemes have been useful in helping improve the quality of analytical data, there needs to be a uniformity in procedure(s) to ensure the mutual recognition of results; a draft harmonised protocol containing guidelines on the organisation of PT schemes is being produced for consideration by ISO. This protocol, however, does not consider the wider issues associated with PT schemes, e.g. their relationship to other aspects of QA.

### 2.2.4.2 Accreditation

Attention has also been directed to the need to ensure quality through the increasing adoption of the principles of laboratory accreditation as customers demand impartial evidence of analytical capability, e.g. UK Accreditation Service (UKAS), formerly the National Measurement Accreditation Service (NAMAS), in conformance with ISO/IEC Guide 25 (ISO, 1978).

This form of accreditation tends to focus on QC matters and includes little about QA of the data, unlike the accreditation obtained under:

- the ISO 9000 and EN 45000 (EN, 1989) series (which relate to quality systems in terms of suppliers of goods and services)
- Good Laboratory Practice, GLP (OECD, 1982) (which is aimed mainly at studies intended to establish chemical risk).

## 2.3 APPLICATION OF AQA TO THE BIOMEDICAL FIELD

### 2.3.1 The Current Issues

Recent years have seen an ever-increasing interest in applying novel materials as prostheses or in medical devices in an attempt to project the biomedical field into a new era. Despite being based on the current understanding of the mechanisms involved in placing synthetic materials in contact with the biological environment of the host tissue, many materials remain unsuccessful.

The many complex interactive biological processes that occur in the presence of an implanted material, and which thereby control its performance, means that there are both limitations and opportunities for misinterpretation during any assessment of this phenomenon. If allowed to remain, the resulting measurement discrepancies will have an even more significant impact on health and financial aspects than is already beginning to manifest itself through problematic biomedical materials and devices that have apparently passed successfully through the existing approval procedures. There have been reported problems associated with the biocompatibility of titanium-coated polytetrafluoroethylene and cobalt–chrome orthopaedic implant materials. Recently silicone breast prostheses have attracted much concern, with punitive damages being awarded. Specific problems exist with the development of biomaterials suitable for use in the clinical field of urology, namely defects in materials for the urinary tract and bladder. There are also ongoing difficulties associated with the development and use of small-diameter synthetic vascular graft materials for cardiovascular surgery. These factors cause the biomedical industry to continue to express concern regarding:

- batch-to-batch variation
- risk assessment of additives, low molecular weight components, degradation products etc.
- the lack of a database of bulk and surface properties, biological safety etc.
- the lack of CRMs.

### 2.3.2 THE PROPOSED APPROACH

It is clear, then, that the valuable traditional approach of sole reliance on the skill and experience of scientists now requires support in order to achieve an independent validated assessment of biocompatibility through:

- the standardisation of manufacturing protocols
- an agreed range of standardised preclinical testing protocols supported by CRMs and accreditation of test laboratories
- performance standards.

These factors tie in closely with the overall guiding principles of the AQA initiative already described. However, the many limitations mean that adoption of the principles of standardised *in vitro* test methods supported by CRMs will not be easy.

Even though the relevant biomedical literature is replete with developed analytical methodologies and the results of applying such methods to particular problems, many of the methods are confined to standard solutions or mixtures and employ simulated rather than real matrix samples, and few of the many results available provide any evidence of their inherent accuracy or QA as the main topic. Comparison of the data is often impossible. Therefore, more standardised *in vitro* test results (combined with those made available through *ex vivo, in vivo* and post-implant evaluation, and/or literature review and subsequent databasing activities) may allow data to be used and compared more effectively, thereby potentially leading to hitherto unseen trends and associated advances in our current knowledge base in this field.

### 2.3.3 EXISTING STANDARD TEST METHODS AND CRMs

As described earlier in this chapter (Section 2.2.2), CRMs can generally be placed within one of two categories:

- as a check on analytical accuracy and precision between laboratories, given the

**Table 2.2**   Selected CRMs available for QC of clinical analysis measurements

| CRM type | Certified parameter |
| --- | --- |
| *Serum and blood* | |
| Human serum | Ca, Mg, Li and progesterone |
| Bovine blood | Cd, Pb |
| Pig kidney | Alkaline phosphatase |
| Human placenta | Creatine kinase |
| *Other matrices* | |
| Human hair | Trace elements |
| *Proteins* | |
| Thromboplastin (bovine/rabbit) | Blood plasma coagulation time |

application of the same analytical procedure(s) (most common in chemical, biological and physical testing laboratories)
• as a means of understanding how the data from a variety of experimental techniques interrelate and describe the system under study (fundamental to the development of new biomedical materials and devices).

To highlight the current lack of relevant CRMs in this type of sector, Table 2.2 shows some of those few CRMs available in perhaps the closest related 'biological' field of clinical chemistry (Colinet, 1992).

However, of more direct concern are the limited quantities of primary polymeric RMs (based on physicochemical characterised low-density polyethylene and filler-free polydimethylsiloxane in sheet and tubular form) which have been proposed in the US for some 10–15 years for use as internal standards for *in vitro* studies of interactions of materials with blood and tissues (Sefton, 1984), and the guidelines for blood–material interactions (NHLBI, 1980a) and physicochemical characterisation (NHLBI, 1980b) of biomaterials. A number of standard tests may also be obtained from the American Society for Testing and Materials (ASTM) and the US Pharmacopoeia (USP).

In the UK, however, there exists only one positive control material (BS, 1991a) and one guideline describing a set of test procedures for evaluating biological hazards (Table 2.3) (BS, 1991b), although a route towards harmonisation was suggested in the tripartite guidance document (involving the UK, Canada and US) (DH, 1986) outlined in the previous chapter.

However, over recent years and in line with the identified requirements of the biomaterials industry, the Laboratory of the Government Chemist (LGC) has been leading the way in undertaking a project and associated collaborative trial aimed at producing a number of relevant CRMs (based on polyethylene, polyvinylchloride and polyurethane matrices) and validated test method protocols for assessing aspects of biocompatibility (particularly cytotoxicity, complement activation and *in vivo* tissue response). Some aspects of this work have now been

**Table 2.3**   UK Guideline BS5736 – Evaluation of Medical Devices
for Biological Hazards

| Guideline parts | |
| --- | --- |
| Part 1 | Guidance for selection of biological methods of testing |
| Part 2 | Tissue implantation |
| Part 3 | Systemic toxicity; Acute toxicity of extracts |
| Part 4 | Intracutaneous reactivity of extracts |
| Part 5 | Systemic toxicity; Pyrogenicity of extracts |
| Part 6 | Sensitisation, delayed contact dermatitis |
| Part 7 | Skin irritation of extracts |
| Part 8 | Skin irritation of solid devices |
| Part 9 | Eye irritation |
| Part 10 | Cytotoxicity of extracts |
| Part 11 | Interactions with blood |

taken up and are being investigated further by a small number of UK university departments. Selected aspects examined by the LGC project have included:

• the development of novel, quantitative immunoenzymatic, cell-specific staining techniques (with computer-aided image analysis) as a valid alternative to the traditional subjective assessment of local tissue response to implanted materials (Vince *et al.*, 1991)
• the establishment of a novel approach for obtaining a quantitative surface energy spectrum/profile (rather than the current single, averaged value) for a material surface as a valid means for providing (in conditions representative of the *in vivo* situation) detailed knowledge, at the molecular level, on the sites and mechanisms involved in events occurring at that surface (Mash, 1992)
• the establishment, standardisation and validation of a novel analytical-scale supercritical fluid extraction/chromatography (SFE/C) method for fingerprinting bulk polymer matrices and for the quantitative extraction and determination (by other common analytical and biological techniques) of their incorporants (Braybrook and MacKay, 1992)
• the development and validation of quantitative *in vitro* assays for assessing the cytotoxicity of bulk materials and their extracts (Braybrook and MacKay, 1992)
• the validation of novel enzyme immunoassay-based kits for evaluating the degree and specific pathway of *in vitro* (human) complement activation induced by specific materials (Maillet *et al.*, 1992).

Through two Commission-funded concerted action projects, EuroBiomat (Lemm, 1992) and part of an ongoing project concerning the long-term performance of biomaterials (Brite-Euram project, BE-7317), some progress has been made on a European front to produce and test potential CRMs using standard test methods. However, neither of the projects followed acknowledged AQA principles, the number of participating laboratories was small, and there was no attempt to introduce 'pass–fail' performance criteria for each test considered (thereby restricting any truly meaningful statistical evaluation). However, the cooperation and integration of harmonisation activities on a European (and international) level has never been more important now that the internal European market for medical devices has been realised, and the 'new approach' Active Implantable Medical Device Directive, AIMDD (90/385/EEC), and Medical Device Directive, MDD (93/42/EEC), described in the previous chapter, are both effective.

Elsewhere internationally, only Japan appears to have reported CRMs and standardised protocols (Tsuchiya *et al.*, 1993).

## 2.3.4 THE WAY FORWARD

Until recently there has been little coordinated European or international effort to bring together and/or develop currently available standardised test protocols and CRMs. As described in the previous chapter, there is now emerging a greater commitment to develop relevant and meaningful European (CEN) and international (ISO) standards, consisting of a number of mutually acceptable protocols for assessing the biological interactions of materials.

CEN has published a range of standards which shadow the work programme of ISO. Associated with these will be the preparation and use of relevant CRMs (ISO, 1996). Although the current Part 12 of the ISO standard correctly acknowledges that there are at present no 'biomedical' CRMs available, it is not limiting in the potential opportunities clearly available. It indicates that there are a number of materials which could prove suitable should they be subjected to proper collaborative trial within Europe, and/or internationally. Some of these could even be materials which have been used for many years and proven successful as prostheses or medical devices. However, these materials tend to be either polymeric, pure metals or metal alloys, and a number of other material types would also be welcomed, e.g. ceramics or stabilised natural tissues. Furthermore, as indicated in the previous chapter, efforts are being directed towards an international interlaboratory comparison exercise, supported by CRMs, in the area of cytotoxicity testing (see also Chapter 6). The aim is to validate specific standard test protocols, with CRMs, for the evaluation of the various end-points and attribute appropriate 'pass–fail' criteria for subsequent incorporation into Part 5 of the ISO standard. This effort is a potential landmark which others will subsequently need to follow. It is therefore essential that all parties play an active role in pursuing these processes and adopting the resulting decisions.

Having proposed an approach to the question of standardisation in the biomedical field, it is worth briefly considering its limitations to the determination of the safety of products, health risks and environmental conditions. Although the approach may lead to improved test methods and result in better accuracy, there will still remain a number of tests which are more subjective in nature where uncertainty remains large (and may continue to do so). For these areas the test methods must be as reproducible and informative as possible, but it may be that their validation needs to take a different route from that generally used. Nonetheless, it is an enormous task to relate any remaining uncertainty of *in vitro* and (animal) *in vivo* test results to an assessment of *in vivo* (human) safety and risk. The required uncertainty must be controlled and matched to the future use of the test results and to economic values involved. This concept is discussed in greater detail in Chapter 11.

## 2.4  CONCLUSIONS

Whatever one's specific views on the complexity of the problem facing the 'biomedical' testing community, it is highly probable that standardisation will remain a necessary component of testing as a basis for better quality products and services well into the next century (albeit perhaps in a form which may differ from that seen today). What is perhaps more certain is the move towards all standardised test methods obligatorily containing statistical data on reproducibility and repeatability of the applied method (already a prerequisite for mandated test methods). However, the achievement of such a goal will require the testing community as a whole to work more closely together at the technical level, prior to the development of relevant standards, during their drafting and also following their publication (in their implementation and continued update). These are therefore both exciting and challenging times.

## 2.5  REFERENCES

Analytical Methods Committee (AMC) (1989) Principles of data QC in chemical analysis. Analyst 114:1497–1503.

Boumans PWJM and Roelandts I (1989) Editorial – News on RMs. Spectrochim Acta 44B:1–3.

Braybrook JH and MacKay GA (1992) Supercritical fluid extraction of polymer additives for use in biocompatibility testing. Polym Intl 27:157–165.

BS (1991a) Poly(vinyl chloride) positive reference material. BSI, Milton Keynes, UK.

BS (1991b) Evaluation of medical devices for biological hazards (BS5736) Parts 1–11. BSI, Milton Keynes, UK.

Cali JP (1975) RMs in clinical chemistry. Fed Proc Fed Am Soc Exp Biol 34:2123–2126.

Cali JP and Reed WP (1976) The role of NBS SRMs in accurate trace analysis. NBS Spec Publ No 422, Washington DC, USA.

Coleman RF (1980) Improved accuracy in automated chemistry through the use of RMs. J Autom Chem 2(4):183–186.

Colinet E (1992) QA in the field of biomedical analysis. Microchem J 45(3):291–297.

DH (1986) Tripartite guidance document for medical devices. Toxicology sub-group of tripartite sub-committee on medical devices, DH, London, UK.

EC (1990) Industrial policy in an open and competitive environment COM(90) 556. EC, Brussels, Belgium.

EN 45000 series (1989) General criteria for the operation of testing laboratories. CEN Central Secretariat, Brussels, Belgium.

Eurachem (1994) Quantifying uncertainty in analytical measurements. Workshop draft, LGC, Teddington, UK.

Garfield FM (1991) QA principles for analytical laboratories, 2nd edn. Royal Society of Chemistry, Cambridge, UK.

Gladney ES, O'Malley BT, Roelandts I and Gills TE (1987) SRMs: compilation of elemental concentration data for NBS clinical, biological, geological and environmental SRMs. NBS Spec Publ 620-111, Washington DC, USA.

Griepink B (1984) Improving the quality of environmental trace analysis. Fresenius Z Anal Chem 317:210–212.

Head AJ (1989) Hierarchy and traceability of CRMs. ISO-REMCO Paper 181, ISO, Geneva, Switzerland.

Horwitz W (1982) Evaluation of analytical methods used for regulation of foods and drugs. Anal Chem 54:67A–76A.

Horwitz W, Kamps LR and Boyer KW (1980) QA in the analysis of foods for trace constituents. J Assoc Off Anal Chem 63:1344–1354.

ISO (1982) Directory of CRM sources of supply and suggested uses. ISO, Geneva, Switzerland.

ISO (1984) International vocabulary of basic and general terms in metrology. ISO, Geneva, Switzerland.

ISO 5725 (1991) Accuracy (trueness and precision) of measurement methods and results: a basic method for the determination of repeatability and reproducibility of a standard measurement method. ISO, Geneva, Switzerland.

ISO Guide 25 (1978) Guidelines for assessing the technical competence of testing laboratories. ISO, Geneva, Switzerland.

ISO Guide 30 (1992) Terms and definitions used in connection with RMs. ISO, Geneva, Switzerland.

ISO Guide 31 (1981) Contents of certificates of RMs. ISO, Geneva, Switzerland.

ISO Guide 34 (1995(E)) Quality systems for RM producers. ISO, Geneva, Switzerland.

ISO Guide 35 (1989(E)) Certification of RMs: General and statistical principles. ISO, Geneva, Switzerland.

ISO TC/102 SC/2 N1004 E (1990) Procedures for statistical evaluation of analytical data resulting from international tests. ISO, Geneva, Switzerland.

ISO (1996) Sample preparation and RMs. ISO TC/194 WG12, Geneva, Switzerland.

IUPAC/ISO/AOAC (1993) Harmonised guidelines for internal QC in analytical chemistry. Draft for 6th Intl Symp, Washington DC, USA.

Lemm W (1992) The RMs of the European Community. Kluwer Academic, Dordrecht, The Netherlands.

Maillet F, Fremeaux-Bacchi V, Uhring-Lambert B and Kazatchkine MD (1992) Assessment of complement activation in clinical samples. J Immunol Methods 156(2):171–178.

Mandel J (1971) Repeatability and reproducibility: a simple analysis providing excellent parameters. Mater Res Mater 11:8–15.

Marchandise H (1987) Accuracy in analyses of biological materials. Fresenius Z Anal Chem 326:613–617.

Marchandise H and Colinet E (1983) Assessment of methods of assigning certified values to RMs. Fresenius Z Anal Chem 316:669–672.

Mash CJ (1992) The surface energy spectrum of PVC. Polym Intl 28:3–7.

NHLBI (1980a) Guidelines for blood–material interactions. NIH Publ No 80-2185, NIH, Bethesda MD, USA.

NHLBI (1980b) Guidelines for physicochemical characterisation of biomaterials. NIH Publ No 80-2186, NIH, Bethesda MD, USA.

OECD (1982) GLP in the testing of chemicals – final report of expert group. OECD, Paris, France.

Parkany M (ed.) (1993) QA for analytical laboratories. RSC, Cambridge, UK.

Parr RM, Muramatsu Y and Clements SA (1987) Survey and evaluation of available biological RMs for trace element analysis. Fresenius Z Anal Chem 326:601–608.

Roelandts I (1989) Biological RMs. Spectrochim Acta 44B:281–290.

Sargent M and MacKay GM (eds)(1995) Guidelines for achieving quality in trace analysis. RSC, Cambridge, UK.

Sefton MV (1984) Chairman's summary: Procurement of primary RMs. Devices and Technology Branch, NIH Publ No 84-1651, Bethesda MD, USA.

Sutarno R and Steger HF (1985) The use of CRMs in the verification of analytical data and methods. Talanta 32 6:436–445.

Taylor JK (1983) RMs: What they are and how they should be used. J Test Eval 11:385–387.

Thompson M and Wood R (1993) International harmonised protocol for proficiency testing of (chemical) analytical laboratories. J AOAC Intl 76(4):926–940.

Thompson M and Wood R (1995) Harmonised guidelines for internal QC in analytical laboratories. Pure Appl Chem 67(4):649–666.

Tsuchiya T, Arai T, Ohkashi J et al. (1993) Rabbit eye irritation caused by wearing toxic contact lenses and their cytotoxicities: In vivo/in vitro correlation study using SRMs. J Biomed Mater Res 27(7):885–895.

Vince DG, Hunt JA and Williams DF (1991) Quantitative assessment of the tissue response to implanted biomaterials. Biomaterials 12:731–737.

# 3

# Biodegradation and Toxicokinetic Studies

DAVID GOTT
Medical Devices Agency, Department of Health, London, UK

## 3.1 INTRODUCTION

Biodegradation and toxicokinetic studies relating to medical devices are expensive, require considerable thought in design and interpretation, and are not undertaken routinely. However, there are some circumstances under which they are essential for risk assessment. The requirement for these studies and the reason why, despite their cost, they can often be economically viable, is discussed in this chapter. Although both types of studies are discussed here, it should be remembered that they are not necessarily linked in practice. This chapter is primarily concerned with the use of these studies in the evaluation of biological safety, although it should be noted that the degradation of materials *in vivo* may actually alter their physical properties and thereby lead to device failure. This may well be catastrophic, but discussion of this is beyond the scope of this book and the standards relating to the evaluation of biological safety; it is, however, dealt with in other international standards, e.g. those being developed by ISO/TC 150.

Meaningful and scientifically valid biodegradation and toxicokinetic studies fit well into the overall evaluation of biological safety by forming the essential link between material characterisation (for which a new ISO/TC 194 work item was accepted in 1996) and the toxicity of material components. The evaluation of biological safety is changing with the ISO 10993 series (outlined in Chapter 1) and EN 1441 from the concept that safety involves passing tests, some of doubtful provenance, to an acceptance of a scientific identification of hazards and estimation of risk in relation to the proposed use.

Current methods may often provide a false sense of security and an unwarranted expectation of safety, the natural consequence of which is a sense of betrayal when an unexpected, untested or even alleged side-effect is observed, for example the recent example of silicone gel, where there is general agreement that the material passes all the tests and yet it has produced enormous concern over alleged

*Biocompatibility Assessment of Medical Devices and Materials.*
Edited by Julian Braybrook. © 1997 John Wiley & Sons Ltd.

adverse effects. However, on a positive note, this experience has led to even more being known about the material, including the realisation that even such a relatively inert material may degrade in the internal milieu of the body (Pfleiderer *et al.*, 1993a,b). Nonetheless, many people find the new approach of hazard and risk analysis intimidating and frightening, as it involves careful assessment and interpretation of data and not just a simple, somewhat unscientific, box-checking exercise. It requires all parties to utilise all available data and to agree on the information needed to fill knowledge gaps. It offers greater scientific validity and, perhaps more importantly, is more ethically beneficial, offering greater reassurance to the public. In view of the public concern over unnecessary animal testing (which often produces meaningless data) and the current national and European legislation, the approach of using fewer, more focused studies also complies with the '3R' principles of Russell and Birch (reduction, replacement and refinement).

## 3.2   DEFINITIONS

Before discussing biodegradation and toxicokinetic studies in detail, it is essential to define some terminology because there is a certain degree of overlap and several common, but different, definitions of toxicokinetics throughout the scientific community. Although there is some overlap between biodegradation and the metabolism portion of toxicokinetic studies, the two can be distinguished based upon the target substrate.

Having discussed the use of toxicokinetics in the way outlined above, a number of kinetic parameters need to be specified. The following definitions are among those agreed in relevant standards:

- 'Absorption' is the process by which an administered substance enters the body. Systemic absorption refers to the amount of test material absorbed into the systemic circulation.
- '$AUC_{0-t}$' is the area under the curve of plasma concentration versus time from time zero to time $t$ following a single dose, where $t$ is normally extrapolated to infinity.
- '$AUMC_{0-t}$' is the area under the curve of first moment plasma concentration versus time from time zero to time $t$ following a single dose, where $t$ is normally extrapolated to infinity, i.e. concentration*time versus time.
- 'Biodegradation' is degradation of components within the body by enzymatic or non-enzymatic reactions, with the formation of byproducts which are not endogenous biochemicals.
- 'Bioresorption' is designed degradation of components within the body by enzymatic or non-enzymatic reactions, with the formation of degradation products which are endogenous biochemicals.
- 'Clearance' is the rate of removal of a compound from the body by metabolism and/or excretion.

- '$C_{max}$' is the maximum concentration of test substance in plasma expressed in mass/unit volume. In another fluid or tissue, the $C_{max}$ should have an appropriate identifier, e.g. $C_{maxliver}$.
- '$C_{maxobs}$' is the maximum observed concentration of test substance in plasma expressed in mass/unit volume.
- 'Degradation product' is the product of bioresorption or biodegradation.
- 'Distribution' is the process by which an absorbed substance and/or its metabolites circulate and partition within the body.
- 'Excretion' is the process by which an absorbed substance and/or its metabolites are removed from the body.
- 'Half life ($t_{1/2}$)' is the time for the concentration of a particular molecular species to decrease to 50% of its initial value in the same body fluid or tissue.
- 'Leachables' are residuals of manufacture (e.g. solvent, monomer) or property-modifying additives that can readily migrate from a material to a physiologically relevant receptor solution.
- 'Mean residence time' is the statistical moment analogy to half-life and provides a quantitative estimate of the persistence of a compound in the body.
- 'Metabolism' is the process by which an absorbed substance is structurally changed within the body by enzymatic reactions. The products of the initial reaction may subsequently be modified by either enzymatic or non-enzymatic reactions prior to excretion.
- '$T_{max}$' is the time at which $C_{max}$ is observed.
- 'Toxicokinetics' is defined here, and in the draft international standard, in line with OECD guidelines on testing chemicals, i.e. it covers absorption, distribution, metabolism and excretion (ADME). (This is essentially identical to the wide definition of pharmacokinetics as applied to drugs; in the pharmaceutical field, toxicokinetics is used to refer to either studies of pharmacokinetics in toxicology studies or studies on pharmacokinetics at concentrations that elicit toxicity, the former being used in industry and the latter in academia. Technically speaking, however, the term used should be 'xenokinetics' but, given the established use of toxicokinetics in the OECD context, this would merely add confusion.)
- 'Volume of distribution ($V_d$)' for a single compartment model is a pharmacokinetic parameter describing the apparent volume which would contain the amount of drug in the body if it were uniformly distributed.

## 3.3 DEGRADATION-RELATED PROBLEMS AND THE NEED FOR BIODEGRADATION AND TOXICOKINETIC STUDIES

The importance of degradation and toxicokinetic studies in the design and development of medical devices can best be indicated through a number of cited examples: silicone gel breast implants, polyurethane-coated breast implants, pacemaker leads, hip implant wear debris, and drug–device combinations.

### 3.3.1 IN VIVO *DEGRADATION OF SILICONE GEL BREAST IMPLANTS*

Interest in the alteration of silicone gel breast implant materials by degradation has arisen as a result of the controversy surrounding these devices. A number of theories have been proposed as a basis for the alleged adverse effects associated with these devices, several of which suggested changes to the structure of silicone that were difficult to reconcile with chemical knowledge.

Studies on the toxicokinetics of silicones can be separated into those based on traditional methods and those utilising nuclear magnetic resonance (NMR) techniques which, although no longer novel, are still uncommon for the study of xenobiotic metabolism *in vivo*. Several reports on the development and use of magnetic resonance imaging (MRI) to identify and locate both ruptured implants and extravasated gel have been published, although the majority of these do not allow firm conclusions to be drawn. A series of reports describe NMR studies on the study of migration and biodegradation of silicone in rats *in vivo* (Pfleiderer *et al.*, 1993a,b; Garrido *et al.*, 1993). They involved both *in vivo* and *ex vivo* studies by both $^1$H and $^{29}$Si NMR for up to 12 months after implantation of silicone gel-filled implants or silicone oil injections. No evidence was shown of silicone in the livers up to 6 months postimplantation of silicone gel-filled implants, but $^{29}$Si spectroscopy and atomic absorption spectroscopy (AAS) showed silicone in the liver and spleen at 9 and 12 months. There was also evidence of the *in vivo* degradation of silicone to hydroxylated silica and highly coordinated silicon products, in both the capsule and liver. Unfortunately, however, there was only limited quantification of silicone metabolism. Despite the high rupture rates at 9 and 12 months (33% and 60% respectively), rupture was only detected on implant removal. These quite elegant data are the first evidence of *in vivo* degradation of silicone materials, although its potentially large significance cannot yet be fully assessed. Furthermore, as the confirmation of the identity of degradation products relies on indirect rather than direct evidence, caution must remain over the interpretation. It is possible that further studies could indicate whether degradation leads to the conversion of silicone to silica (despite unfavourable thermodynamics) and, if so, its extent, thereby allowing greater elucidation of this putative mechanism of action.

### 3.3.2 POLYURETHANE-COATED BREAST IMPLANTS

Polyurethanes are polymers containing the urethane group commonly formed by reacting an aromatic or aliphatic isocyanate with a polyfunctional alcohol, typically a polyether- or polyester-based diol. Either hard or soft segments, which are more or less resistant to chemical degradation and determine the mechanical properties of the polymer, may be formed. Examples of hard segments include aromatics, cycloaliphatics or aliphatic diisocyanates, with diols or diamines as chain extenders. Examples of soft segments include low molecular weight (MW) hydroxy-terminated polyethers or polyesters. All polyurethanes are, to a greater or lesser degree, susceptible to hydrolysis of the urethane bond, with production of low MW fragments. However, polyesterurethanes are further susceptible to hydrolysis of the ester linkages, with initial production of low MW fragments and final production of the components of the polyester diol. The ether linkages in polyetherurethanes are more resistant to such cleavage and may be essentially hydrolytically stable in the absence of other factors. The predominant reaction depends on local chemical groups, stereochemistry, polymer morphology and pH of the local environment. Local pH is decreased by ester hydrolysis and could accelerate urethane hydrolysis. Degradation is particularly accelerated in the presence of metal ions and mechanical stress (Williams, 1995).

The polyurethane used in the manufacture of breast implants is a polyester-urethane manufactured from polyethylene glycol adipate (PEGA) and toluene diisocyanate (TDI) (Equation 3.1). The latter comprises a mixture of 2,4-TDI and 2,6-TDI isomers in a 4:1 ratio. TDI is unstable in aqueous environments and reacts to form the equivalent toluenediamine (TDA) isomers.

**Equation 3.1**

$$HO\{(CH_2CH_2O)_kCO(CH_2)_4COO(CH_2CH_2O)_k\}_mH + OCN(C_6H_3Me)NCO$$

$$(PEGA) \qquad\qquad\qquad (TDI)$$

$$[O\{(CH_2CH_2O)_kCO(CH_2)_4COO(CH_2CH_2O)_k\}_mCONH(C_6H_3Me)NHCO]_x$$

$$(Polyesterurethane)$$

Cross-linking of the polymer chains is achieved by incorporating a triol form of PEGA. Added water reacts with residual isocyanate to release TDA and carbon dioxide, which produces the foamed product. TDA readily reacts with isocyanate groups to form imide bonds. The amount of residual TDA should theoretically be low, although detectable amounts (around $0.1\ \mu g/g$) have been shown to be present in foam direct from the chemical manufacturer. This residual TDA should be removed by washing during fabrication of the foam for breast implant use.

Release of TDA from polyurethane foam requires cleavage of two adjacent urethane bonds and, although this has been reported for the polyesterurethane foam coating of breast implants, it has not been reported in polyetherurethanes. In vitro hydrolysis of polyurethanes has been shown to produce the corresponding diamines under extreme conditions, 90% TDA yield being obtained with water at 160–200°C for 6 hours. Most tested polyurethanes showed MW changes after 4 hours in water at 120°C, the rate and extent of polyesterurethane degradation being higher than that of polyetherurethanes (probably as a result of their lower hydrolytic stability and an autocatalytic effect on ester and urethane bond cleavage of the carboxylic acid groups formed). The polyesterurethane foam from breast implants has been shown to degrade in vitro after several hours in alkali (0.3–3 M sodium hydroxide, NaOH) at 37°C, yielding up to 17% TDA. Even the use of more physiological conditions still resulted in degradation. These findings have been supported by more recent *in vitro* studies, although the possible breakdown of extractable oligomers during some analytical procedures indicates that estimates of foam degradation from some earlier studies may need to be treated with caution. Equally, the possible underestimation owing to the limited aqueous solubility of TDI derivatives must be borne in mind. However, the best estimate of foam degradation from *in vitro* studies suggests an annual rate of 1%, i.e. equivalent to *ca.* 2 mg 2,4-TDA from typical polyurethane-covered breast implants.

The *in vivo* degradation of subcutaneously implanted [14]C-labelled polyurethane foam has been studied in rats over 56 days. The [14]C-labelled TDI was incorporated during foam synthesis, although there were few details of either its position or specific activity. From 15 mg of foam, implanted at two sites, urinary excretion of radioactivity was detected as *ca.* 0.9% and faecal excretion 1.2%, but the metabolites could not be identified. There was little activity in tissues after 56 days, although no data were presented either on the implantation site or total recovery. The majority of studies have utilised histological methods to demonstrate disappearance or fragmentation of the foam from the implantation site, although this has been shown potentially to be an artefact in the preparation of the histological sections (Szycher and Siciliano, 1991). The apparent fragmentation seems to arise from ingrowth of tissue into the foam structure and sections being cut through the 3D matrix of the foam. This work did, however, demonstrate *in vivo* degradation of the foam, leading to decreases of at least 30% over a 9-year period. There is now both direct and indirect evidence for the breakdown of the polyurethane foam used on 'Même' and 'Replicon' breast implants *in vivo*, not only in animals but also in humans. Again 2,4-TDA is produced. The rate of breakdown is not accurately known, although an apparent half-life of 23 months (which appears to fit other reported observations) would suggest that the majority of the exposure arises in the first 4–5 years postimplantation.

The toxicokinetics of 2,4-TDA have been studied in rats and mice after intraperitoneal administration and in rats, rabbits and guinea pigs after oral administration. The majority of the dose (90%) was excreted in urine after both oral and intraperitoneal administration, except for one study with intraperitoneal administration where 22% was excreted in faeces between 6 and 16 hours postadministration. Peak tissue levels were observed at 1 hour after intraperitoneal administration. The toxicokinetic data indicate that acetyl and other acid-labile conjugates, e.g. monoacetyl derivative, diacetyl moiety, ring hydroxylation products, and both the oxidation of the benzylic methyl group and its acetylated product, are the main metabolites of TDA in rat and man. Little unchanged 2,4-TDA was excreted after oral administration in rats, although free 2,4-TDA has been shown in the urine of women with polyurethane foam-coated breast implants. Elimination appears to be biphasic, with half-lives of 2–5 hours for the rapid phase and more than 6 days for the slow phase. The possibility that plasma levels and elimination may be affected by the acetylator phenotype cannot be discounted, although the available data are insufficient to indicate whether rapid or slow acetylators are the greater risk. Rapid acetylation of TDA *in vivo* may ameliorate exposure to the parent compound, but the possibility of a significantly different toxicokinetic situation by slow acetylation cannot be discounted. This effect may result in different risks of 2,4-TDA in these two populations, a carcinogenic risk arising from exposure to 2,4-TDA from polyurethane-covered breast implants. It is difficult to estimate the extent of such a risk from the current data, but the possibility that the risk is greater in tissues close to the implant than systemically cannot be discounted.

### 3.3.3 POLYURETHANE PACEMAKER LEADS

Two principal degradation mechanisms, metal-catalysed oxidative degradation and environmental stress cracking, are prevalent in polyurethane pacing leads and lead to failure of its insulation properties. It is interesting that both seem to be required in this material. In contrast to the polyurethane-coated breast implants, there is little or no evidence for the release of significant amounts of degradation products from the leads, and hence little concern over their risks. However, degradation modifies the polymer chain and affects its mechanical properties. The failure associated with this degradation is outside the scope of a biological safety evaluation but within that of implant properties in the risk assessment, and indicates the need for some common methodology in both areas.

### 3.3.4 HIP IMPLANT WEAR DEBRIS

A similar situation to that observed with polyurethane pacing leads exists with hip implant wear debris. Debris formation appears generally to be due to mechanical wear, which again is outside the scope of the ISO 10993 series. However, the assessment of the risks associated with this wear debris, which represents a biological hazard, requires an evaluation in line with the principles of ISO 10993-1. It should be remembered that there may also be chemical degradation accompanying the mechanical wear.

### 3.3.5 DRUG–DEVICE COMBINATIONS

Drug–device combinations, which here include the incorporation of growth factors and other biological modifiers (as well as traditional pharmaceuticals) into devices, e.g. antibiotic-containing bone cements, necessitate toxicokinetic studies. The use of such studies must be the key link in establishing the safety and efficacy of the active ingredient in the device combination, with the data establishing its acceptability as a pharmaceutical under medicinal product regulations. In the absence of a detailed toxicokinetic evaluation the safety of the device cannot be demonstrated under these circumstances. Both systematic and local risks associated with the levels of the active material need to be evaluated.

## 3.4  THE VALUE OF TOXICOKINETIC INFORMATION

A brief description of the absorptive process in the gastrointestinal tract can be used to highlight how existing knowledge from several fields (including toxicokinetics) can be used to evaluate hazards, thus rendering additional studies unnecessary. This can be applied to other routes in an equivalent manner, e.g. the lack of volatility of amalgam components (other than mercury) at body temperature means that effects related to vapour exposure in industrial uses can be dismissed as not relevant to the proposed use.

The absorption barrier in the intestine can be considered as a number of possible rate-limiting barriers comprising the bulk fluid in the lumen, the aqueous unstirred boundary layer, the glycocalyx and acid microclimate, the apical membrane of the absorptive cell, cell contents, basal membranes and intestinal blood flow. There are five possible routes of absorption. Transcellular and paracellular passive diffusion is the principal mechanism for absorption of nutrients and xenobiotics; facilitated diffusion and active transport are specialised mechanisms for uptake of important ions and nutrients, e.g. L-dopa uptake by aromatic amino acid carriers; and endocytosis is of importance in the absorption of lipid micelles and is implicated in the uptake of macromolecules, particles and peptides. The latter uses the lymphatic system for transport to the bloodstream and, although quantitatively this route is of relatively minor importance, it is believed to have a major role in certain specialised functions.

The major physicochemical determinants of absorption are partition coefficients (lipophilicity), solubility and dissociation constants. Molecular size also affects absorption and is determined by a hybrid of MW and structure. The pathophysiological factors include rate and pattern of gastric emptying, rate of intestinal transit, thickness of the aqueous unstirred layer, intestinal blood flow, luminal and microclimate pH, and metabolism in the lumen and wall. The formulation factors include binding to macromolecules, micelle formation, dissolution rate, particle size and chemical stability.

Absorption requires that a molecule cross the membrane of the intestinal cell principally by passive diffusion. The tight junctions between the intestinal cells are considered to be impervious to cations with MWs $> 300$ Da. The limitation for anions is unclear, as the acid microclimate may effectively exclude these from the sites. The most important basic principle of absorption remains the pH partition hypothesis, which requires that a xenobiotic be in solution at the surface of the membrane and possess sufficient lipid solubility to dissolve in the hydrophobic inner layers of the membrane. The state of ionisation of a compound is a major factor influencing this lipid solubility, with the non-ionised species of an ionisable molecule being preferentially absorbed. It has become increasingly clear, however, that the pH partition hypothesis is only a partial explanation of the mechanism of drug absorption, as there is evidence of absorption of some highly hydrophilic molecules (even with partition ratios up to 30:1 in favour of the aqueous phase) and molecules which are ionised at the pH of the intestine (e.g. quaternary ammonium compounds). There have been several attempts to modify the pH partition hypothesis to accommodate these anomalies, the most useful being the concept of aqueous pores, although there is some debate as to whether these are actual or hypothetical constructs to explain the data. It has been suggested that highly hydrophilic compounds could reach sufficient concentration in the aqueous unstirred layer to partition into the membrane, from which they would rapidly move to the aqueous environment inside the cell and hence provide the concentration gradient to drive diffusion. There has also been recent evidence of apparent binding sites for some ionised molecules, which are then absorbed as non-ionised complexes.

The majority of knowledge about the effect of physicochemical parameters on absorption derives from studies across series of related drug moieties. Plots of absorption rate ($\log K_a$) against partition coefficient ($\log P$) show a general increase until a plateau value is reached at $\log P$ values of 3.5–4. The absorption rate for isolipophilic compounds varies by factors up to 20, illustrating the difference between different series of compounds. A plot of absorption rate against aqueous solubility for the same series of compounds would show a decrease to a plateau value approaching zero. The superposition of these two curves usually results in absorption rate maxima around $\log P$ values of 2.5–3.5 for a particular series of compounds. The influence of MW lies in its role in determining molecular size which influences diffusivity within a solvent. There is usually little influence at MWs $< 500$–600, where solubility, the dissociation constant and the partition coefficient are major determinants. The effect on absorption begins to become important at MWs of 500–1000; it is almost impossible to be more precise, as molecular structure and shape are also important determinants in this range. It is unlikely that there will be significant absorption by passive diffusion of the majority of compounds with MWs $> 1000$; there will be some minimal absorption (*ca.* 1–2% of the ingested material) by more specialised routes, e.g. peptides and macromolecules, and highly lipophilic compounds in micelles. Thus a MW of 1000 could be regarded as a threshold for practical purposes, although the use of estimates of molecular shape could permit the setting of priorities at $< 1000$, especially when solubility and the partition coefficient data are also considered (*ca.* $< 600$). Thus for polymeric materials used in the gastrointestinal tract, e.g. in enteral feeding tubes, it would not be necessary to evaluate the systemic toxicity of polymer and oligomers, whereas lower MW additives might require a detailed evaluation.

## 3.5 DEGRADATION EFFECTS AND EVALUATION

The degradation of medical devices and materials in the biological environment is of particular relevance because the degradation products may have different behaviours from the bulk material in terms of biological response, and they may also affect device or material properties.

Degradation products can be generated in different ways, either mechanically (by relative motion between two or more different components), by release from the surface (due to interactions with the environment) or through a combination of the two. Mechanical wear causes mostly particulate debris, whereas the release of substance from surfaces due to leaching, breakdown of structures or corrosion can lead to free ions or reaction products in the form of either reactive or stable organic or inorganic compounds. Agglomerations of larger quantities of stable degradation products may, however, have physical effects on the surrounding tissues. Degradation products may remain at the site of their generation or may be transported within the biological environment by a variety of mechanisms. The level of their biological acceptance depends on their nature and concentration, and has been assessed widely through clinical experience and particular studies. For well described and clinically accepted degradation products no further investigation may be necessary, whereas for new and unknown degradation products relevant testing must be carried out, the approach to their assessment varying with the nature of the material under investigation.

### 3.5.1   EFFECT OF DEGRADATION PRODUCTS ON THE BODY

The effects of degradation products on the body can only be assessed on a case-by-case basis. The major concern is the potential for formation of reactive products, e.g. 2,4-TDA (as discussed above). The production of a reactive chemical can lead to adverse effects, and the nature of these will determine the actual risks involved. A more detailed examination of risk analysis is discussed in Chapter 10, but the formation of even small amounts of a genotoxin may be a significant risk, whereas similar amounts of a non-genotoxin may pose little or no risk.

The interaction of wear particles with tissues can provoke a vastly different response to their parent material, partly owing to their greater surface area, but also to the different surface properties of the materials. Methods of material surface analysis are therefore important. A detailed discussion of techniques applicable to polymeric biomaterials is given in the next chapter. Thus the possibility of degradation should always be considered when undertaking a risk assessment, and its influence documented. For most devices this will be fairly easy, as the degree and type of exposure will obviate the need for any further consideration.

### 3.5.2   EFFECT OF DEGRADATION PRODUCTS ON DEVICE OR
### MATERIAL PROPERTIES

In addition to effects on the body, the degradation products can also affect the device or material properties. The degradation of one or more materials in a device can lead to loss of integrity and even functional failure, e.g. pacemaker leads. This can only be assessed for a particular device during its design and risk assessment. The consequences of such failures would, at a minimum, probably lead to reoperation (which is itself classified as serious injury) and, at worst, death. These aspects lie beyond the scope of ISO/TC 194, but are addressed by ISO/TC 150. However, there is a need to maintain an effective relationship between these committees in order to ensure a common evaluation of potential consequences: it would be patently absurd to have a vastly different, non-physiological degradation method indicating intrinsically unlikely hazards.

### 3.5.3 THE INTERNATIONAL TECHNICAL REPORT ON DEGRADATION

During the course of their initial work, WG2 of ISO/TC 194 believed it was premature to specify degradation methods in a standard, but they did publish a technical report (TR 10993-9) describing the current state of the art. Although this report was undoubtedly worthy, it was flawed in ways which detracted from its usefulness and undermined its credibility and validity. It was perceived as uncertain in its purpose and intended audience. The document made no attempt to clarify whether or not the suggested tests should be performed at all times for all devices, thus leaving the reader with the impression of a requirement for overtesting. There was no discussion of the possible effects, validity and data interpretation resulting from testing samples with surfaces which would not normally be exposed in use. The principles behind the analysis of substances and materials in body tissues/fluids should have been described in greater detail. Guidance on areas such as number of samples, repeatability, calibration curves, assay validation etc. should also have been provided, while recognising that the actual assays need to be developed on a case-by-case basis. The exclusion of high-performance liquid chromatography (HPLC) and newer methods, e.g. supercritical fluid extraction/chromatography (SFE/C), from the cited analytical methods was equally worrying.

As a result of the above factors, ISO/TC 194 WG 2 believed that most progress could be made by developing a standard on toxicokinetics (WG 13 was subsequently formed for this task) and working on more specific test methods for three classes of materials, namely polymers, metals and ceramics. These are intended to provide more detailed conditions for degradation studies on these materials and decision criteria on their necessity. All of these documents are gradually progressing, although the lack of input from sufficient experts is an additional burden to their production.

## 3.6 CURRENT EUROPEAN AND INTERNATIONAL STANDARDS

### 3.6.1 THE INTERNATIONAL STANDARD ON TOXICOKINETIC STUDY DESIGN

The draft ISO standard (10993-16) sets out when to consider evaluation of toxicokinetics and stresses the need to design these studies on a case-by-case basis as required for risk assessment. The principles to be incorporated in the study design are outlined, with guidance being provided on the detailed aspects which need to be considered in individual studies. This guidance is based on the large amount of published literature which exists on the methodologies and techniques utilised in toxicokinetic studies on chemical entities, particularly pharmaceuticals and pesticides (since these are largely independent of the intended use of the chemical entity).

### 3.6.2  THE EUROPEAN STANDARD ON DESIGN OF DEGRADATION STUDIES

CEN/TC 206, under mandate, recently established a WG to produce a draft standard on the design and need for degradation studies. The objective is to develop this draft into a standard through ISO/TC 194. The document is analogous in concept to the draft international standard on toxicokinetic study design, in that it sets out when to consider such evaluations, the need to design studies on a case-by-case basis and the principles to be incorporated in the study design. However, it also emphasises the initial use of a theoretical assessment of potential degradation products, which may be sufficient for risk assessment. Thus this standard gives a framework for the systematic evaluation of the potential and practical biodegradation of medical devices, and the design and performance of biodegradation studies.

## 3.7  DESIGN OF STUDIES

### 3.7.1  GENERAL CONSIDERATIONS

As already noted (Sections 3.4 and 3.5), both degradation and toxicokinetic studies can be a vital part of the testing strategy in a scientific evaluation of biological safety. Although it is not possible to devise a testing strategy without evaluating and interpreting data, this particular issue is outside the scope of this chapter. The need to carry out supplementary evaluations, or to consider initial evaluations not suggested in ISO 10993-1 for a particular use, requires a decision based on knowledge and informed speculation. This is particularly true for studies which cannot be justified on ethical and economic grounds in every case. The decision to undertake such studies must be based on the need for this information for risk assessment. The evaluation of the need to perform specific studies will make use of knowledge from other studies or similar materials which may provide sufficient reassurance in a particular case.

Thus any experimental study used in the evaluation of biological safety should be designed on a case-by-case basis and should not simply follow a 'cookbook' approach which may lead to critical aspects being ignored. The greatest reassurance that can be provided to consumers is derived from an open-minded evaluation of hazards and their associated risks. It has been said that a little thought and a soupçon of chemical knowledge would have stopped the choice of the particular polyesterurethane used on polyurethane-coated breast implants and avoided the associated public concern over an unnecessary risk. It must be remembered that the degree of reassurance required varies with the intended purpose and the likelihood of a readily foreseeable misuse; it would be pointless to require the same level of data for a material in transient contact with skin as for an implanted material.

A study protocol must be written prior to commencement of the study. In this protocol methods need to be defined to the greatest extent possible; it is not possible to specify precise methods in advance in studies which require empirical development of analytical methods, e.g. metabolite isolation. The study report must include all the information necessary to evaluate the results, and study quality and validity. The application of good laboratory practice (GLP) principles to biological tests is essential. If data quality in reports is poor, or details are omitted, then it is not possible for the data to be independently evaluated and they are essentially useless, whether the chemical or material involved poses a risk or not. These internal quality checks may be the only means available for regulatory bodies to have confidence in the data. The importance of this approach has already been discussed in principle (see Chapter 2), but it is even more important in toxicokinetic and degradation studies as it also reinforces the confidence of third parties in the decisions reached in the analytical phases of these studies. Reports on the biological safety of medical devices often contain no details on the sex, age or body weight of the animals used, justifying this on the grounds that 'these are not specified in the appropriate method'. Although these parameters are not always relevant to the choice of animals for a study, this information may be important for interpretation and must be specified in the report. At its worst it is often not even clear that animals of the same sex or similar age were used in the test or control group, although it is hoped that this is due to nothing more than poor-quality reporting. The lack of diet or water analysis is often justified because 'there were no contaminants suspected that could interfere with this study'. Frequently, too, no evidence is cited in support of such sweeping statements, the absence of which compromises the reported data and clearly breaches the OECD Mutual Acceptance of Data Agreement and GLP requirements.

The draft standards on degradation and toxicokinetic study design make it crystal clear that testing is expected to be relevant under specific circumstances. For degradation studies these are when:

- substantial quantities of a potentially toxic or reactive substance may potentially be released
- the device is being designed to be bioresorbable
- the device is intended to be implanted for a long period and significant biodegradation is expected.

For toxicokinetic studies these are when:

- a constituent or degradation product of the device or material is present in concentrations which may produce adverse effects at the rate of release available for uptake
- the device is being designed to be bioresorbable
- the device is intended to be implanted for a long period and significant biodegradation or corrosion is known, or likely, and/or migration of significant quantities of a leachable from the device/components occurs.

### 3.7.2 CEN WORKING DRAFT ON DEGRADATION STUDIES

There is the potential for hazards to arise from the degradation of a medical device and its components, so that the probability of intended and unintended degradation of the materials needs to be evaluated and documented. The CEN draft document recognises that a consideration of this potential is essential to the evaluation of the safety of a device.

Information on the chemistry of the component materials is considered in the light of the intended use of the device, and includes the identification of constituent chemicals and known degradation products. As already stressed above, the standard makes clear those conditions for which the study is appropriate and those where it is neither necessary nor practical for all medical devices, namely when:

- substances which have the potential to leach out or be released have a history of safe clinical use in the achieved or expected quantities and rates from the particular device
- sufficient degradation data relevant to the substances and degradation products already exist.

It is valuable to begin with *in vitro* studies, both for animal welfare reasons and also to determine probable, rather than possible, degradation products. The need for *in vivo* studies can be determined by the results of these initial studies.

The draft suggests that, as a minimum, the study protocol defines the methods by which chemical and physicochemical properties, surface morphology and biochemical properties are to be investigated, the rationale being that the extent and rate of release of degradation products depends on their concentration at the surface, migration to the surface within the material, solubility in the physiological milieu, and on the flow rate of the physiological milieu. These practical degradation studies shall be performed according to appropriate GLPs.

The analytical methods have to be fully described in the study report and must be able to detect and characterise degradation products in the study media. The description in the report will include details of the validation of the assay methods. These analytical methods must be specific, sensitive, reproducible and linear over a range of expected analyte concentrations. The document emphasises that the test report must be complete, and provides an '*aide mémoire*' of information to be included when relevant. This typically should consist of:

- a description of the material and/or device being investigated for degradation, e.g. chemical composition, and processing, conditioning and surface treatment(s)
- an assessment of degradation
- an identification of degradation products, e.g. form and condition of degradation products
- a description of the test methods, conditions, materials and operating procedures
- a statement of compliance with GLP
- a summary interpretation and discussion of the results.

There is also guidance on how to conduct and document a theoretical evaluation of degradation. Again, information on the device, its constituent components and materials and its intended application is essential, and these must be described and considered in evaluating degradation. The potential for both intended and unintended degradation of the materials need to be included. This involves identification and characterisation of possible mechanisms of degradation, identification and characterisation of known, probable and potential degradation products, and a summary of this evaluation. Part of the evaluation is the assessment of the necessity for and the extent of experimental biodegradation studies. Appropriate additional experimental studies are considered when essential information regarding the degradation of a device or the biological effects of the potential degradation products is missing from the theoretical evaluation. Clinical experience, existing investigations, published data and analogies with known devices, materials and degradation products may allow adequate evaluation of the biodegradation of a device. The evaluation may be completed or complemented by appropriate experimental degradation studies, if necessary, followed by biological tests. An overview of different classes of materials and typical related degradation mechanisms and degradation products is currently incorporated in the draft, but this is intended to be neither exhaustive nor to act as a checklist.

The above assessment could lead to the conclusion that sufficient data are available, so that further studies are not necessary, and this would be documented in the risk analysis. Alternatively, the primary assessment will lead to the conclusion that additional experimental degradation studies are necessary. Some informative references to relevant standards are given alongside the principles for designing and reporting these studies. If degradation products require biological evaluation, then a documented biological assessment in accordance with the principles of EN 30993-1 is to be conducted.

## 3.7.3  TOXICOKINETIC STUDIES

### 3.7.3.1  Background

The potential hazard posed by a medical device may be due to the interactions of its components or their metabolites with the biological system. Medical devices may contain leachables (e.g. residual catalysts, processing aids, residual monomer, fillers, antioxidants, plasticisers, degradation products) which migrate from the material and have the potential to cause adverse effects in the body. A large amount of published literature exists on the use of toxicokinetic methods for other chemical entities, and the methodologies and techniques utilised in such studies form the basis of the guidance on study design in this draft ISO standard.

### 3.7.3.2 Leaching Studies

It is possible to provide reassurance on leachables based on historic data, although differences in agreement relating to the approach required do not help mutual recognition of data. In order to provide this level of reassurance it can be argued that data on leachability should be collected under worst-case conditions. Then, in circumstances where these conditions raise concern over the degree of migration of a particular compound, realistic studies would also be carried out. On the other hand, the reverse situation can be argued, although there must remain doubt that sufficient reassurance can be provided as realistic studies can easily be biased by their heavy reliance on the assumptions of the 'real' situation.

Knowledge of the identity and total quantity of the leachables is also required, but the provision of satisfactory results from such studies may be sufficient for risk analysis, thereby obviating the need for toxicokinetic or degradation studies *per se*.

The end-use of the device often does not appear to be considered in the design of extraction studies. The use of static extraction conditions, despite the fact that usage involves fluid (blood) flow through the device, is a common flaw. There is increasing evidence that movement across the surface of a material can significantly increase the extraction of components from that material. Studies from the Laboratory of the Government Chemist using agitation methods have demonstrated a 1000-fold difference in extraction. Suffice it to say, therefore, that the extraction methods should be relevant to the proposed use as a minimum, and prudence would again suggest that a worst-case scenario is desirable to increase reassurance.

Without evidence that migration to the extractant occurs under the extraction conditions used, and that these are appropriate to the proposed use, the requirement for leaching studies is not scientifically valid.

### 3.7.3.3 ISO Standard on Toxicokinetic Studies

Toxicokinetic studies are again designed on a case-by-case basis. A study protocol is written prior to the commencement of the study, defining the methods to be used, e.g. dosing and sample collection. The results of leaching studies are considered to determine the appropriate method for toxicokinetic studies. Again, information on the chemical and physicochemical properties, surface morphology and biochemical properties is essential.

Analytical methods able to detect and characterise leachables and metabolites in biological fluids and tissues are defined in the study protocol as far as possible. These methods should be specific, sensitive, reproducible and linear over the range of expected analyte concentrations, and validation of the assay method is again presented in the report. It is recognised that the performance of toxicokinetic studies of mixtures is often difficult: it may be preferable to undertake toxicokinetic studies with the characterised chemical entity that has the potential to be toxic, rather than with an extract of the material. The study design must state the physiological fluid, tissue or form of excreta where analyte levels will be determined. The possibility of analyte binding to tissue, circulating proteins or red cells, or the sample (e.g. amount and affinity) should be contained in the report; it should also be demonstrated that this does not lead to underestimation of analyte concentration. Blood is convenient to sample and thus is often the fluid of choice for kinetic parameter and absorption studies. It is necessary to specify whether the analysis is carried out on whole blood, serum or plasma, and this choice must be validated. There should be sufficient data points collected, with adequate spacing to allow determination of kinetic parameters; in theory this should cover several terminal half-lives, although in practice the constraints of the analytical method will often necessitate a compromise.

## 3.8  GUIDANCE ON TEST METHODS

### 3.8.1  GENERAL CONSIDERATIONS

Studies should be performed in an appropriate sex and species of animal. Healthy young adults should be acclimatised to laboratory conditions for at least 7 days. They should be transferred to individual metabolism cages, when used, for a further acclimatisation period of at least 24 hours. The environmental conditions should be as recommended in animal welfare guidelines for the test species. During the study, conventional animal food and drinking water should be freely available unless otherwise specified in the protocol. Animals should be randomly selected into groups for each time period studied; group sizes of at least three for small animals and at least two for larger species should be used. At the appropriate specified sacrifice times animals should be humanely killed.

A non-radiolabelled compound may be utilised, provided that suitable validated assay procedures exist for the compound in the relevant samples and that the metabolism of the compound is well characterised. If necessary, the test substance should be radiolabelled in a metabolically stable position, preferably with $^{14}$C or $^3$H, and be of a suitable radiochemical purity ($>97\%$). When using $^3$H the possibility of exchange should be considered. The radiolabelled compound should be diluted, when appropriate, with non-radiolabelled substance. The specific activity and radiochemical purity of the test substance must be known and reported.

The test substance should be administered by an appropriate route; this should be relevant to the use of the medical device, but the study design may require the inclusion of other routes for comparison. The test substance should be prepared in a suitable sample appropriate to the route of dose administration. The stability of the sample under the proposed conditions of administration should be known and reported.

In dose balance studies, animals should only be housed in metabolism cages. Urine and faeces should be collected at low temperature (or in the presence of preservative) to prevent postelimination microbial modification. Blood for whole-blood or plasma analysis should be collected in the presence of a suitable anticoagulant. Wherever possible, controls should be collected prior to dosing. In some studies collection of controls (e.g. tissues) from the test animals is not possible and these should be obtained from a control group. Collection times should be appropriate to the type of study being performed. For studies involving excreta this is usually 24-hour periods over at least 96 hours. Where blood sampling is required, blood is collected according to a specified schedule ranging from minutes to hours over a period of 24–72 hours. Toxicokinetic studies should be performed according to GLP.

The test report shall include the following information, where relevant:

- the strain and source of animals, environmental conditions, diet, age, sex etc.
- test substance and sample purity, stability, formulation, amount administered
- test conditions, assay methods, extraction and detection methods, means of validation, tabulation of individual results at each time point, overall recovery of material
- tabulation of individual results at each time point
- GLP compliance statement
- discussion and interpretation of results.

## 3.8.2  SPECIFIC GUIDANCE

### 3.8.2.1  Kinetic Parameters

A number of kinetic parameters can be determined depending on the design of the study. These include absorption rate, elimination rate, AUC, half-life, volume of distribution, clearance, mean residence time and AUMC. It is not necessary to determine all kinetic parameters in every study: the aim is to provide the necessary information for risk assessment. Kinetic parameters can only be determined for a particular molecular species, and hence the assay must be specific and sensitive to that molecular species. True kinetic parameters of a relevant compound can only be determined following intravenous (i.v.) administration, and it may be necessary to include such a limited study in the design of kinetic parameter studies. This allows the fraction of the dose absorbed to be calculated and serves as a correction in estimating parameters in other studies. A number of computer programs exist for estimating kinetic parameters and the software should be validated prior to use and this validation documented. The assumptions entered into the program and the choices in modelling should also be documented. Sampling is normally more frequent in the early phase of absorption and elimination, although samples need to be obtained over as much of the elimination phase as possible (ideally 3–4 half-lives) to provide the best estimates of kinetic parameters. The major determinant is often assay sensitivity.

### 3.8.2.2 Absorption

Absorption is dependent on the route of administration, the physiochemical form of the chemical, and the vehicle of administration. It can be estimated from blood, serum and tissue concentrations. Complete bioavailability studies may be considered. The choice of the appropriate type of study depends on the other information required, the availability of radiolabelled material and the assay method. In a kinetic parameter study, the absorption rate constant can only be estimated reliably only if sufficient samples are taken in the absorption phase. Well-characterised and validated *in vitro* methods exist to estimate gastrointestinal and percutaneous absorption, the latter only being validated when the stratum corneum is the rate-limiting barrier.

### 3.8.2.3 Distribution

Distribution studies generally require a radiolabelled compound. Quantitative studies determining levels in tissues or whole-body autoradiography studies for qualitative or semiquantitative determination should be performed. In general, sampling times in distribution studies are $C_{max}$, 24 hours and 168 hours or longer, depending on compound elimination. Intermediate times may be used when these additional data are required.

### 3.8.2.4 Metabolism

The metabolism cages should permit separate collection of urine and faeces throughout the study. For studies of up to 14 days the urine and faeces should be individually collected at 24 hours and then every 24 hours until the end of the experiment. In some study designs animals may be sacrificed at intermediate times. Samples may be collected prior to 24 hours where it is probable that the test substance or its metabolites will be rapidly excreted. For studies of longer duration sampling over the initial period should occur as for the short-term studies, but thereafter samples should be obtained for a continuous 24-hour period per assessment period. The use of metabolism cages for prolonged periods may be detrimental to animal welfare, and hence sample collection at the later times in such studies involves taking representative discontinuous samples and extrapolating these to continuous sampling. The carcasses and/or target organs of the individual animals should be retained for analysis and blood collected for analysis of whole blood and plasma concentrations. After collection of the samples from the metabolism cages at the time of sacrifice, the cages and their traps should be washed with an appropriate solvent. The resulting washes can be pooled and a representative fraction retained for analysis. The recovery of material should be $100 \pm 10\%$ when radiolabelled materials are used. The amount of compound in each fraction should be analysed by suitably validated procedures for either radiolabelled or non-radiolabelled material in the appropriate milieu. Where radiolabelled material is concerned total compound and metabolites are assessed, unless a specific assay is used. If the radiolabelled compound cannot be sufficiently recovered in the excreta or in the body, collection of expired air should be considered. The recovery range specified is that usually intended; this may not be achievable in all cases, and reasons for any deviation should be stated and discussed in the report. Levels of radioactivity in the biological milieu should be determined, e.g. by liquid scintillation counting, although it must be stressed that this represents a mixed concentration of compound and metabolites, and no kinetic parameters can be derived from it. Where isolation of metabolites is considered necessary this may involve a number of chromatographic procedures (e.g. HPLC, thin-layer chromatography (TLC), gas–liquid chromatography, GLC) and extractions, and the resulting material should be characterised by a variety of both chemical and physical techniques (e.g. mass spectrometry, NMR). The use of tissues, cells, homogenates and isolated enzymes for the study of metabolism *in vitro* is well documented, but these methods identify potential metabolism which may not occur *in vivo* unless the compound is available at the appropriate site.

## 3.9  CONCLUSIONS

As already indicated, although the future for both European and international standards on degradation and toxicokinetic studies is assured, with their role in the biological evaluation of safety being vitally important, there is still much to be done. Current discussions relating to chemical characterisation (already discussed briefly in Chapter 1) are also pertinent, and can only place further importance on the issues which have been addressed here.

## 3.10  REFERENCES

Garrido L, Pfleiderer B, Papisov M and Ackerman JL (1993) *In vivo* degradation of silicones. Magn Reson Med 29:839–843.

Pfleiderer B, Ackerman JL and Garrido L (1993a) *In vivo* localised proton NMR spectroscopy of silicone. Magn Reson Med 30:149–154.

Pfleiderer B, Ackerman JL and Garrido L (1993b) Migration and biodegradation of free silicone from silicone gel-filled implants after long-term implantation. Magn Reson Med 30:534–543.

Szycher M and Siciliano AA (1991) Polyurethane-covered mammary prosthesis: a nine year follow-up assessment. J Biomat Applic 5:282–322.

Williams D (1995) Polyurethane paranoia: flexible friend or deadly foe. Med Dev Tech April:7–10.

# 4
# The Surface Analysis of Polymeric Biomaterials

MARTYN DAVIES, C.J. ROBERTS, S.J.B. TENDLER AND
P.M. WILLIAMS
Department of Pharmaceutical Sciences, University of Nottingham

## 4.1 INTRODUCTION

The surface chemistry of biomaterials plays a major role in determining host response and biocompatibility. Protein conditioning and cellular adhesion phenomena on exposure to body fluids have been linked directly to the surface energetics and morphology of materials (Absolom et al., 1984; Schakenra et al., 1984; Andrade, 1985a; Missirlis and Lemm, 1991; Horbett and Brash, 1995). Some of the key problems in biomaterial performance can be related directly to surface interactions, e.g. the encrustation of urinary stents is mediated through inorganic deposits forming on an adsorbed protein layer derived from urine. The level of bacterial adsorption and colonisation in implant-associated infection is also dependent in part on the surface structure (Wilcox, 1993). The interfacial chemistry of polymeric colloids intended for site-specific delivery in vivo plays a major role in determining the avoidance of uptake by Kupffer cells within the liver, thereby ensuring the extended circulation times necessary for organ-selective targeting (Illum and Davis, 1987; Davis et al., 1993). Many more examples exist in the literature in all areas of the exploitation of biomaterials. In recognition of the importance of interfacial chemistry, considerable efforts have been made to tailor the surface properties of biomaterials to optimize in vitro and in vivo performance while retaining the desired bulk properties. A wide range of thin-film technologies, from sophisticated self-assemblies and protein arrays to facile polymer overcoating, have been exploited to either minimise surface interactions or promote highly selective molecular recognition. Such methodologies have been utilised in all forms of biomedical devices, ranging from implants, stents and advanced delivery systems through to biosensors and immunolattices.

In order to gain a greater understanding of the structure–activity relationships that exist between biomaterial surfaces (and their possible modification) and

*Biocompatibility Assessment of Medical Devices and Materials.*
Edited by Julian Braybrook. © 1997 John Wiley & Sons Ltd.

observed biointeractions, a range of advanced surface analytical techniques have been exploited over the last 20 years or so to define the interfacial properties. As our knowledge has deepened through the use of these methodologies, it is evident that we must not assume that the surface chemistry of a biomedical device is similar to that of the bulk phase. Phase separation or preferential surface orientation of one or more components, or the presence of contaminants derived from the fabrication process, are just some of the factors which will manipulate the surface chemistry of biomaterials. The interfacial region is also a dynamic structure where the influence of hydration and adsorption of biomolecules on exposure to body fluids may induce significant surface structural reorganisation.

The purpose of this chapter is to examine what are believed to be the *major* methods that can provide valuable information on, primarily, the biomaterial surface chemical structure, topography and, briefly, surface interactions. Although there are a number of surface analytical methodologies available (Andrade, 1985b; Riviere, 1990; Walls, 1990; Sabbatini and Zambonin, 1993), this chapter concentrates on those believed to have the maximum impact in biomaterial interfacial characterisation. This selection is a personal perspective of the authors and does not detract in any way from the value and quality of information derived from other methods. By drawing from the key developments within the literature, the potential and limitations in the ability of the methods to define the surface properties of biomaterials for both fundamental studies and biomaterial device development will be illustrated and, where appropriate, fruitful areas for future exploitation suggested.

## 4.2   SURFACE CHEMICAL ANALYSIS

There are a number of chemical analysis techniques for defining the surface structure of materials (Andrade, 1985b; Ratner, 1988; Riviere, 1990; Walls, 1990; Sabbatini and Zambonin, 1993). This section focuses on the two that are proving to be the most suitable for the chemical analysis of the solid polymeric biomaterials, namely X-ray photoelectron spectroscopy (XPS) and secondary ion mass spectrometry (SIMS).

### 4.2.1   XPS AND SIMS: THEORY

There are many detailed discussions of the theoretical principles and practical applications of the SIMS and XPS techniques (Briggs and Seah, 1990, 1992; Beamson and Briggs, 1992; Vickerman and Briggs, 1996), and therefore only the salient features will be highlighted here.

In the SIMS experiment (Figure 4.1a), a surface is bombarded by a primary beam of noble gas ions or atoms (eg $Ar^+$, $Xe^+$, $Ar^o$) under ultrahigh vacuum (UHV) conditions. These primary particles penetrate the surface to a depth of around 30–100 Å. The kinetic energy of these particles is dissipated in the form of

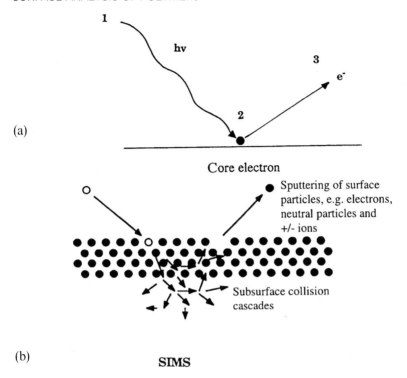

**Figure 4.1**  Simple schematic diagram of XPS and SIMS analysis. (a) XPS; 1: specimen irradiated with low-energy X-rays; 2: X-rays cause photoionisation of atoms in specimen; 3: response of sample (photoemission) observed by energy spectrum of emitted photoelectrons. (b) SIMS

a collision cascade. At some point remote from the site of impact this cascade causes the emission of neutral particles, electrons, and positively and negatively charged ions. These elemental or molecular cluster ions are analysed in terms of their mass to charge ratio, yielding positive and negative secondary ion mass spectra.

The operating conditions for SIMS experiments on organic and inorganic surfaces are now well defined (Briggs *et al.*, 1984; Briggs and Hearn, 1985; Brown and Vickerman, 1986) where the practical mass range extends from m/z 0–800 for quadrupole instruments to m/z 0–10 000 for time-of-flight (ToF) machines, and the mass resolution of the latter can reach to the order of 5–10 000 for routine experiments. It has been shown that the ions detected within the SIMS analysis arise from a sampling depth of around 10Å under normal 'static' experimental conditions, underlining the high surface sensitivity of the technique (Hearn *et al.*, 1987; Lub and van Velzen, 1989). The interpretation of these spectra can yield substantial structural information on surface chemistry by exploiting the expertise and knowledge gleaned from conventional mass spectrometry rules (McLafferty and Turecek, 1993). There are, however, a number of problems

**Table 4.1**   Key facts on XPS and SIMS analysis of polymers (adapted in part from Zhuang and Gardella, 1996)

|  | XPS | SIMS |
|---|---|---|
| Incident particles | X-rays | Ions/atoms (Ar, $Xe^+$, $Ga^+$) |
| Emitted particles | Photoelectrons | Secondary sputtered ions |
| Environment | UHV | UHV |
| Nature of information | All elements except Li | All elements/isotopes; molecular ions |
| Depth of analysis | 1-5 nm depending on incident x-ray angle | 1 nm for polymers |
| Resolution | 0.5 eV | Dependent on quad. or ToF instrument; quad. *ca.* 1 m/z ToF mass resolution $10^3$ |
| Sampling area | 5 $\mu$m–10 mm | 5 $\mu$m–10 mm |
| Lateral resolution | 5 $\mu$m | sub-$\mu$m |
| Detection levels | 1%; monolayer | ppm; elements 0.01%; molecular monolayer |
| Instrumentation cost | Expensive ( > £250K) | Expensive ( > £250K) |
| National service centres | Yes | Yes |

associated with the SIMS analysis of materials, particularly organic surfaces. The major drawback is that the ion yields vary with surface composition, known as 'matrix effects', leading to problems in quantifying SIMS data (Briggs and Seah, 1992). This may be overcome to some extent by the use of ratios of ion intensities within each spectrum (Lub *et al.*, 1987; Briggs and Ratner, 1988; Davies *et al.*, 1988b, 1991), but this is only semiquantitative at best.

In the basic XPS experiment (Figure 4.1b), the sample surface is irradiated by a source of low-energy X-rays under UHV conditions (Andrade, 1985b; Briggs and Seah, 1990; Riviere, 1990; Walls, 1990; Beamson and Briggs, 1992; Sabbatini and Zambonin, 1993). The incident photons interact with core-level electrons (i.e. those not involved in bonding) in the surface atoms and photoionisation takes place. The resultant photoelectrons possess a kinetic energy described by Equation 4.1.

**Equation 4.1**

$$K_E = h\nu - B_E - f$$

where

$K_E$   is the kinetic energy of the emitted photoelectron,
$h\nu$   is the X-ray photon energy,
$B_E$   is the binding energy of the electron in its atomic orbital,
$f$   is the work function of the spectrometer surface.

The emitted electrons are collected by an electrostatic energy analyser and detected as a function of the kinetic energy. The corresponding binding energy of each core electron is characteristic of the atom to which it is bound, and the XPS spectrum thus allows identification of all elements except H and He, e.g. the C1s and O1s photoelectrons appear at *ca.* 285 and 530 eV. In contrast to SIMS, the elemental composition of the surface may be quantified by measuring the peak areas for each of the element signals within the spectrum and normalising these values using sensitivity factors which reflect the probabilities of the different orbitals interacting with an X-ray photon (Briggs and Seah, 1990). Even though the core electrons are not involved in chemical bonding, any change in the valence environment will result in a change in their binding energy. Thus, deconvolution algorithms are employed to determine these binding energy shifts within the elemental binding energy envelope, providing valuable quantitative function group analysis of the surface, e.g. C-F, $C-F_2$ and $C-F_3$ environments may be clearly resolved within the C1s envelope as they lie at *ca.* 287.9, 290.9 and 292.69 eV, respectively. The sampling depths of the XPS may be varied from 10 to 100 Å for polymers through the use of different angles of incidence for the X-rays.

The relative merits of the two techniques are highlighted in Table 4.1.

It has become clear that the two methods provide complementary information where the XPS analysis delivers quantitative elemental and functional group data and SIMS allows a greater insight into the molecular structure and organisation of the interface. The following section will illustrate how these two techniques may be employed in tandem for the characterisation of biomaterials.

## 4.2.2  XPS AND SIMS: ANALYSIS OF POLYMERIC BIOMATERIALS

### 4.2.2.1  Polymer Spectral Analysis

There is a well-established literature on XPS and SIMS analysis of polymeric systems, including those designed for biomedical applications (Ratner, 1988, 1993, 1995; Davies and Lynn, 1990; Feast *et al.*, 1993). To illustrate the rich vein of information gleaned from their application to polymers, the surface chemical analysis of the biodegradable polymer 75:25 poly(DL lactide-co-glycolide), PLGA, widely exploited in a range of different biomedical applications, is discussed in depth.

Figure 4.2 shows the survey XPS scan of a PLGA film (Davies *et al.*, 1988b, 1989; Shard *et al.*, 1996) where the C1s and O1s are clearly evident at *ca.* 285 and 530 eV.

An analysis of the peak areas shows that the percentage carbon and oxygen content compares well with the theoretical stoichiometry of the copolymer C:O, 1.38:1. Previous analysis of PLA and PGA homopolymers (Davies *et al.*, 1989) found that three specific carbon environments achieved the best fit in the deconvolution of the C1s envelope at 285, 287.1 and 289.4 eV. By reference to standard databases within the literature, these binding energies were shown to correspond to the C-C/C-H, C-O-CO (ester) and O-C = O (carboxyl) environments respectively within the monomer structure. The percentage compositions of these components of the C1s are indicated in Figure 4.2. The results are in excellent

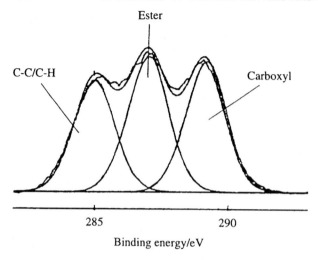

**Figure 4.2** XPS analysis of 72:25 poly(DL lactide-co-glycolide), PLGA, film (Davies *et al.*, 1989)

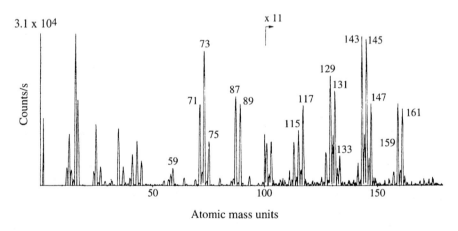

**Figure 4.3** Negative ion SIMS spectrum of 72:25 PLGA film (Davies *et al.*, 1989)

quantitative agreement with the hydrocarbon:ester:acid carbon atom ratio of 3:4:4 deduced from the molecular structure of 75:25 PLGA.

The PLGA negative ion SIMS spectrum is presented in Figure 4.3.

Analysis of PLA and PGA homopolymers using SIMS and the copolymer data represents essentially an overlay of the individual PLA and PGA homopolymer spectra, but with some important additional ions. A classic feature of the SIMS analysis of polymers is the presence of ions whose mass is diagnostic of the intact or fragments of the monomer unit, and in many cases the functional groups or side-chains present within the monomer structure. This is clearly illustrated in

Figure 4.3, where it can be seen that many of the ions observed directly correspond to either of the monomers within the PLGA polymer chain. Anions corresponding to PLA monomer repeat units (-CH(CH$_3$)-COO-) or M$_{LA}$, where M is the molecular weight of the PLA monomer, are observed for (nM$_{LA}$ $\pm$H)$^-$ at m/z 71/73 and 143/145 and also for (nM$_{LA}$ + O $\pm$ H)$^-$ at m/z 87/89 and 159/161, where $n$ = 1–2. Similarly, ions derived from the PGA monomer unit (-CH$_2$-COO-) or M$_{GA}$, are seen at m/z 59 and 115/117 for (nM$_{GA}$ $\pm$H)$^-$, and at m/z 73/75 and 131/133 for (nM$_{GA}$ + O $\pm$H)$^-$ where n = 1-2. In addition there are a number of peaks within the negative ion spectra which do not correspond to homopolymer fragments, such as m/z 129 and 147, which may be assigned to the anions (M$_{LA}$M$_{GA}$-H)$^-$ and (M$_{LA}$M$_{GA}$+OH)$^-$ arising from random sections of the polymer sequence. A similar series of cations is observed in the positive ion SIMS spectrum of the PLGA copolymer (Shard et al., 1996).

The complementary nature of the XPS and SIMS analysis is quite clear from the above example. The XPS data provide excellent quantitative elemental and functional group information. The appearance of high-sensitivity and high-energy resolution instruments is increasing the degree of structural information and confidence in deconvolution analysis of core-level shifts. A number of standard databases now exist where full spectral information is available for an extensive range of polymer types (Beamson and Briggs, 1992). The analysis of the PLGA polymer illustrated the detailed molecular data provided by SIMS, allowing the determination of the monomer structure and copolymer composition and, as noted above, details of the copolymer sequence. Despite the fact that such mass spectra can seem daunting, a number of reviews and reference databases are now available to aid the novice and the experienced operator alike in spectral interpretation (Feast and Munro 1987; Feast et al., 1993; Davies and Lynn, 1990; Briggs and Seah, 1992; Benninghoven and Rading, 1994; Vickerman and Briggs, 1996; Zhuang and Gardella, 1996). There has been considerable focus on the mechanisms of the fragmentation patterns observed and debate on the assignment of structures. A number of approaches have been developed to assist in the identification of ion structures. The derivation of surface functionalities (Chilkoti and Ratner, 1993), the use of isotopic labelling of one or more portions of the repeat unit (Briggs and Munro, 1987; Lub et al., 1987; Brinkhaus and van Ooij, 1988), the exploitation of MS-MS (Leggett et al., 1990a,b, 1992) (i.e. producing a daughter ion mass spectrum of a dominant ion within a parent mass spectrum) have all aided the determination of ion structures and contributed to our knowledge of polymer fragmentation patterns. However, it is the advent of ToF instruments with working mass resolutions of around 10 000 that has made the significant advance in ion assignments and which is currently the gold standard for SIMS analysis.

The quantification problem is a severe limitation of the SIMS technique. The influence of matrix effects on ion yields has been noted and has limited direct quantitative information from individual ion intensities. However, many examples now exist in the literature where authors have correlated ratios of ion intensities diagnostic of the monomers within a copolymer with bulk composition to derive semiquantitative data (Lub et al., 1987; Briggs and Ratner, 1988; Davies et al., 1988b, 1991; Weng et al., 1995). Figure 4.3 shows the ratio of $89/89 + 75$ against bulk LA composition for a range of PLGA copolymers where 89 is diagnostic anion of LA, i.e. $(M_{LA} + OH)^-$ and 75 is the corresponding anion for GA, i.e. $(M_{GA} + O \pm H)^-$. A linear relationship is observed, which suggests that the changes in the surface structure reflect the changes in bulk composition across the copolymer series. Similar studies have been performed on a wide range of copolymeric systems including poly(etherurethanes), poly(alkyl methacrylates), poly(orthoesters) and many other polymer classes. Such semiquantitative relationships have been exploited in deriving sequence information from copolymers from methacrylate series (Briggs and Ratner, 1988) and also from PLGA systems where the SIMS data were able to provide an indication of their block vs random nature (Shard et al., 1996).

### 4.2.2.2  XPS and SIMS: Applications to Characterisation of Polymeric Biomaterials

The surface chemistry of polymer biomaterials may not be representative of that in the bulk phase. Surface segregation, phase separation, modification and contamination will all lead to a modification in the interfacial chemistry and hence, potentially, to changes in the nature of the biointeractions observed. XPS and SIMS have been applied to defining the surface chemistry of a range of biomedical systems. Selected examples are discussed below, but the wide range of applications is illustrated in Table 4.2.

SIMS and XPS have a major role in defining the surface chemistry of complex polymeric interfaces where phase separation and segregation may occur, e.g. the relative surface dominance of hard and soft segments of polyurethanes has been the subject of much debate in the literature (Ratner, 1988). SIMS and XPS studies have extended the understanding of the influence of bulk polymer composition on the presence of phase-separated domains within polyurethane surfaces (Hearn et al., 1987, 1988; Briggs and Seah, 1992; Yoon et al., 1994), a phenomenon which is thought to have implications for their biological activity. Surface studies have revealed that the interface is composed of a mixture of hard and soft domains, rather than one component forming an overlayer (Figure 4.4).

Another area where the surface segregation of polymer end-chains plays a vital role in the performance of biomaterials is in the formation and stability of polymer colloids for diagnostics, imaging and advanced delivery applications. Combined SIMS and XPS studies have played a significant part in understanding the structure–activity relationships between surface end-group (Figure 4.5) (Davies et al., 1993a) and copolymer composition (Davies et al., 1994, 1996) in terms of classic colloid characterisation measurements and in interpreting in vivo biodistribution for a range of standard and biodegradable materials (Dunn et al., 1994; Brindley et al., 1995).

**Table 4.2** Examples of the potential application areas for XPS and SIMS characterisation of biomedical materials

| | Application areas |
|---|---|
| Material surface chemistry | Phase separation – PUs (Hearn et al., 1987, 1988; Yoon et al., 1994).<br>Surface end groups – polymer films (Linton et al., 1996) and colloids (Davies et al., 1993a).<br>Surface cross-linking in gels (Chilkoti et al., 1993b).<br>Hydration of surface (Lewis and Ratner, 1993; Lin et al., 1993).<br>Surface functional group derivatisation (Chilkoti and Ratner, 1993; Alexander et al., 1996).<br>Stereoregularity (Zimmerman and Hercules, 1994).<br>Oligomers; analysis (Blestos et al., 1985) and at polymer surfaces (Reichlmaier et al., 1995).<br>Copolymer sequence formation (Briggs and Ratner, 1988; Shard et al., 1996).<br>Blend composition (Lhoest et al., 1995b).<br>Amphilic networks (Park et al., 1995). |
| Surface modifications | Structural re-organisation (Lewis and Ratner, 1993; Lin et al., 1993; Magnani et al., 1995; Shard et al., 1995).<br>Ion bombardment (Lhoest et al., 1995a).<br>UV irradiation (France et al., 1995).<br>Plasma polymerisation – e.g. PHEMA, PS, methacrylate films (Castner et al., 1993; Chilkoti et al., 1993a; Lopez et al., 1993; Leggett et al., 1995; Ward and Short, 1995).<br>Plasma modification – PS by different gases (Petrat et al., 1994a,b).<br>Immobilised polymers – sterically stabilised colloids (Brindley et al., 1995) and non-fouling coatings for implants (Sheu et al., 1993).<br>Immobilised biomolecules – proteins (Griffith et al., 1996), lipids and oligonucleotides (Patrick et al., 1994) on sensors; saccharides (Davies et al., 1993b; Sugiyama and Oku, 1995) and lipids (Sugiyama et al., 1993) on colloids; and proteins on implants (Leute et al., 1994).<br>Surfactant adsorption – quantitative isotherms (Batts and Paul, 1994) and non-fouling coatings (Bridgett et al., in press).<br>Contamination – lubricating agent and PDMS (Feast and Munro, 1987); plasticisers (Davies and Lynn, 1990; Briggs and Seah, 1992); and residual surfactants (Koosha et al., 1989; Weng et al., 1994). |
| Biomolecule surface chemistry | ✓Protein structure (Mantus et al., 1993; Dombrowski et al., 1996).<br>✓Protein adsorption (Gilding et al., 1980; Subirade and Lebugle, 1994; Baty et al., 1996; Davies et al., 1996) and quantitation (Muddiman et al., 1996).<br>Drug and peptide delivery systems (Garbassi and Carli, 1986; Davies and Brown, 1987; Davies et al., 1988a; John et al., 1995). |

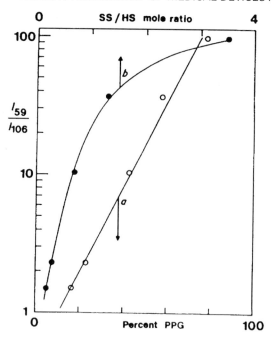

**Figure 4.4**    The log ($I_{59}/I_{106}$) SIMS peak intensity ratio plotted as a function of bulk concentration of polyetherurethane (containing polypropylene glycol, PPG, in the soft segment) in terms of (a) the % PPG content, (b) the ratio of soft segment:hard segment. The cation m/z 59 is a characteristic fragment of PPG, whereas m/z 106 is characteristic of the hard segment. Although the surface is clearly enriched with soft segments, hard segments may still be detected even at the highest PPG levels. This suggests that previous overlayer surface models of polyurethane interfaces need to be reconsidered

A wide variety of approaches are being employed to surface engineer the interface of biomaterials to achieve optimum biocompatibility while leaving the desired bulk properties unchanged. It is important to define the nature and level of the changes in surface chemical environment to interpret the alteration in surface energy which will modify the level of cellular and biomolecular interactions. One of the most important areas for the application of SIMS and XPS analysis has been in characterising the level of surface modification for a wide variety of techniques, from the plasma modification/polymerisations to the surface grafting of biomolecules and polymers at interfaces. For example, in Figure 4.6 the surfaces of contact lenses subject to oxygen plasma discharge treatment were shown to change from an organosiloxane-dominated polymer surface to a surface silica phase (Fakes *et al.*, 1988).

Numerous other examples exist in studying the influence of production conditions on the complex surface chemistry of plasma-modified (Petrat *et al.*, 1994a,b) or polymerised films (Castner *et al.*, 1993; Chilkoti *et al.*, 1993a; Lopez

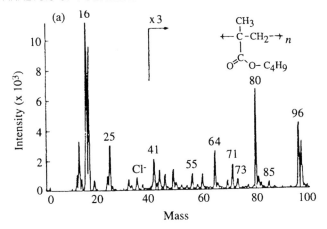

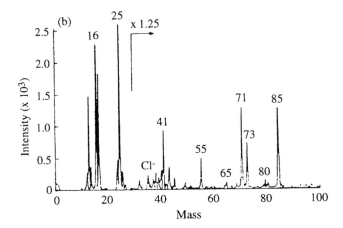

**Figure 4.5** The negative ion SIMS spectrum of (a) polybutylmethacrylate latex (m/z 0–100); (b) polybutylmethacrylate latex dried and cast from chloroform. The sulphate polymer end-groups responsible for stabilising the colloid surface dominate the spectrum in (a) at m/z 64, 80 and 96. After disruption of the colloid interface by dissolving in solvent (b), the sulphate levels are very low and the peaks diagnostic of the methacrylate backbone and ester butyl sidechain at m/z 55/85 and 71/73, respectively, now dominate. This provides clear evidence for enriched levels of polymer end-groups at the colloid surface

*et al.*, 1993; Leggett *et al.*, 1995; Ward and Short, 1995). In contrast to such processes, which can yield multiple surface functionalities, the careful surface grafting of a monolayer of biomolecules such as proteins/phospholipids or polymers has been explored to improve the compatibility of implants and also to act as templates for immunosensors. Again, SIMS and XPS have been shown to provide valuable information (see Table 4.2) on the level of surface immobilisation

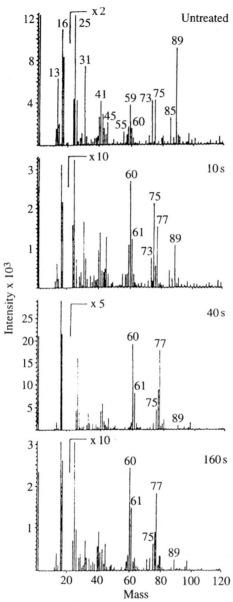

**Figure 4.6**   Negative ion SIMS spectra of untreated and oxygen glow discharge-modified contact lens surfaces. The surface transforms from an organosiloxane-dominated interface (e.g. m/z 89 corresponding to $OSi(CH_3)_3^-$) to inorganic silica functionalities (e.g. m/z 60/61 corresponding to $SiO_2^-/SiO_2H^-$) with treatment time

(Ferruti *et al.*, 1982; Davies and Lynn, 1990; Leggett *et al.*, 1993; Leute *et al.*, 1994; Hagenhoff, 1995) and surface segregation (Davies *et al.*, 1993b; Lin *et al.*, 1993; Sugiyama *et al.*, 1993; Sugiyama and Oku, 1995). Angular XPS studies also provide an opportunity to probe below the top molecular layers of a modified surface, e.g. the polymer chemistry beneath a protein film, to define the composition of what is now frequently termed 'buried interface' (Tyler *et al.*, 1989).

The techniques also have a significant role in detecting the presence of inclusion/adsorbed molecules at or within the polymer surface (see Table 4.2). XPS provides an indication of the presence of the molecules within the interface by deviation from the known atomic ratios for the polymer or the appearance of a diagnostic element not present in the polymer structure. Many of the low molecular weight inclusion molecules yield distinctive fragmentation patterns within the SIMS experiment, including intact molecular ions and/or dominant diagnostic ion fragments. Early examples included the determination of drug molecules within the surface of polymeric delivery systems (Garbassi and Carli, 1986; Davies and Brown, 1987; Davies *et al.*, 1988a; John *et al.*, 1995). More recently, the differentiation between different proteins adsorbed to polymeric substrates has been described using a multivariate analysis of ToF–SIMS spectra (Mantus *et al.*, 1993). Such an approach can be employed to study the presence of surface contaminants, e.g. silicone oils, catalysts, surfactants etc. Again, XPS revealed the high level of surface contamination in materials used as international standards (Ratner *et al.*, 1993). The presence of a lubricating agent, bis-ethylene stearamide, responsible for the surface properties of commercial poly(etherurethane), Pellothane, has been identified by SIMS (Feast and Munro, 1987). SIMS and XPS analysis have also played a key part in the detection of residual surfactants on colloid surfaces and the evaluation of subsequent cleaning methods (Koosha *et al.*, 1989; Weng *et al.*, 1994).

### 4.2.2.3 The Hydrated State – UHV Compatibility?

One of the major concerns in studying polymeric interfaces using SIMS and XPS is the effect on the interfacial chemistry on exposure to UHV during the analysis (Swalen, 1987). Such materials may exhibit surface reorganisation to minimise the interfacial free energy on exposure to a different environment (Lewis and Ratner, 1993). Surface restructuring may occur on contact with an aqueous milieu, particularly for complex materials, where elements of the macromolecular structure may have different hydrophobicities and compatibilities. This phenomenon may be exacerbated by the adsorption of proteins and cells at this interface. A number of workers have developed a method to study the mobility and restructuring of the outermost surface region of a polymer in an XPS and SIMS experiment using cryogenic sample preparation techniques to preserve the integrity of the hydrated surface structure (Lewis and Ratner, 1993; Gardella, unpublished results). The potential of this approach was shown by the study of the hydrated and dry surface of a triblock polymer based on the hydrophilic

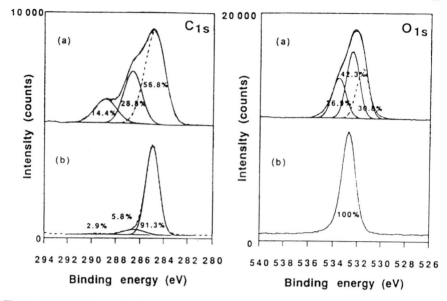

**Figure 4.7** High-resolution C1s and O1s XPS spectra for HEMA grafted on to silastic elastomer after (a) hydration, freeze drying and analysis at $< -120°C$; (b) raising the sample temperature to 25°C and vaccum drying *in situ*. The dramatic differences in both C1s and O1s between the two samples is very evident. The hydrated surface is estimated to be composed of *ca.* 95% HEMA. In contrast, the dehydrated surface has undergone dramatic rearrangement to a surface composition of 90% silicone

poly(hydroxyethylmethacrylate), PHEMA, and the hydrophobic poly(*n*-octyl-styrene), POS (Ratner, 1995). In the dry state the surface is completely dominated by the POS portion of the polymer, whereas in the hydrated environment the hydrophilic polymer PHEMA is the major component at the interface. Hence the analysis of certain complex materials using SIMS and XPS must be undertaken with care, and on the understanding that a different surface may be reacting to the exposure to a complex biological locale. Such studies have already provided some sense of the timescales and depth of reorganisation that may occur, and this appears a very fruitful area for future investigations in biomaterial surface chemistry.

### 4.2.3 CORRELATIONS OF SURFACE CHEMICAL ANALYSIS DATA WITH BIOLOGICAL INTERACTIONS

The relationship between surface structure and interfacial chemistry is well known and is thought to have a major impact on the nature and extent of biological interactions at polymeric interfaces. For example, SIMS and XPS provided crucial information in terms of interpreting the relationship between the level of surface-grafted poly(ethylene oxide) PEO chains and the *in vivo* biodistribution of a range of advanced drug delivery colloids prepared with

**Table 4.3**  Examples of the potential value of the correlation of XPS and/or SIMS data with biological interactions

---

Platelet interactions with PEU composition (Hanson *et al.*, 1982).
Human vein endothelial cells on PS culture surfaces and RF-plasma modified PTFE (Steele, 1995).
*In vitro* leucocyte adhesion to plasma-modified PU surfaces (Bruil *et al.*, 1994).
Surface determinants of neuronal survival and growth on self-assembled monolayers (Stenger *et al.*, 1993).
Substrate hydrophilicity on epithelial cell adhesion (Dewez *et al.*, 1996).
Adhesion and spreading of human skin fibroblasts on gradient surfaces (Ruardy *et al.*, 1995).
*In vitro/in vivo* studies on PHEMA-grafted membranes in artificial cornea development (Lee *et al.*, 1996).
Correlations between surface properties and blood conpatibility of PE/PVA blends (Klee *et al.*, 1996).
*In vitro* cell responses to differences in PLA crystallinity (Park and Cima, 1996).
Cell adhesion controlled by ion implantation of polymer (Lhoest *et al.*,1995).
Circulation time and organ uptake of surface modified colloidal delivery systems (Dunn *et al.*, 1994), (Brindley *et al.*, 1995).
Bone cells on PS surfaces (Callen *et al.*, 1993).

---

different PEO surface densities (Illum and Davis, 1987; Davis *et al.*, 1993) (Figure 4.7).

Although there have been a number of such studies which correlate surface data with some feature of biointeractions at the cellular and protein level, it must be recognised that both the complexity of the substrate chemistry and the nature and kinetics of the biological processes have limited the resolution of unifying hypotheses. Ratner summarises this issue rather well: 'The lack of information on the controlling variables for surface processes is as much related to the difficulty in quantifying meaningful biological processes as it is with the measurement and interpretation of surface analysis data'. Clearly much work is needed here to translate all the innovation and industry in accumulating high information surface chemical data in the interpretation of biological responses to biomaterials. With greater availability of instrumentation, and with national facilities emerging, publications featuring both surface biophysical and some *in vitro/in vivo* data are becoming more commonplace. A number of excellent studies now exist in the literature and a selection is highlighted to illustrate the potential in Table 4.3.

A number of points deserve further comment. There is a clear need to carefully consider the method of information analysis in extracting meaningful correlations when faced with the mass of biophysical and biological data. In this respect, an interesting example is the use of multivariate statistics in establishing the most important surface chemical variables derived from SIMS, XPS and contact angle measurements in the adsorption of fibrinogen to a range of polymer surfaces (Perezluna *et al.*, 1994). The models were able to determine the relevant data from complex information derived from the SIMS analysis which related to fibrinogen adsorption. Based on the information from the polymer series studied, the authors also showed that, with care, the statistical methods employed were able to accurately predict the adsorption behaviour on other materials.

Many fundamental studies rely on the choice of suitable standard materials of defined wettabilities to probe biological interactions (Andrade, 1985a). Clearly, XPS and SIMS have a role in ensuring the quality (even contamination) of these standard materials. Several workers have advocated the use of gradient surfaces with continuously varying surface chemical composition (as measured by XPS) to study cellular responses to material surface properties (Elwing, 1987; Ruardy et al., 1995). Such an approach is argued to yield more convincing conclusions than the use of a range of differing materials with different wettabilities. Other workers are turning to self-assembled monolayers as well-defined substrates (e.g. with -CH$_3$, -OH, -NH$_2$ terminated) to glean further information on structure–activity relationships for biological–surface interactions (Mrksich et al., 1995; Leggett and Downes, in press).

### 4.2.4  SUMMARY

The preceding sections have highlighted the potential of surface chemical analysis in defining the interfacial chemistry of wide range of biomedical materials and devices. The technology is maturing and the community is gaining a greater understanding of the value of the information gleaned from exploiting such advanced instrumentation. The techniques can play a major role within the biomaterials industry in the development of new systems and in the evaluation of their performance. However, it is apparent from this article that, although the methods have many advantages, there are a number of limitations, and clearly a number of key issues require further attention. Used in isolation, the data may lead to false interpretation; however, when employed within a portfolio of analytical, biochemical and in vivo studies they provide much added value and make a major contribution to the development of a new generation of biomaterials.

## 4.3  SURFACE MORPHOLOGY AND TOPOGRAPHY

Surface morphology and topography are determined by the material's physicochemistry and processing, and are likely to feature in the host response to a foreign material. A number of standard approaches are available to characterise the surface texture, including electron microscopy. This section will focus on the use of one of a new generation of microscopes, the atomic force microscope (AFM), which features the imaging of native biomaterials within an aqueous environment to a high resolution, thereby allowing the study of dynamic interfacial events of importance in biomedical science.

### 4.3.1  INSTRUMENTATION

A number of excellent reviews have been published in the literature describing

AFM instrumentation and operation (Binnig, 1992; Overney *et al.*, 1992; Burnham and Colton, 1993; Marti and Amrein, 1993; Hansma *et al.*, 1994; Quate, 1994), and therefore only the salient features will be summarised here.

In the AFM experiment a three-dimensional map of the material surface is produced from the forces of interaction between the surface and a sharp probe, which is rastered or scanned across the interface. The forces of interaction may be attractive or repulsive, and these are exploited in the different modes of operation described later. The basic design of AFM is shown in Figure 4.8.

In practice, the probe commonly consists of a silicon nitride pyramid with a sharp tip (radius 20 nm) suspended from a flexible silicon cantilever with a defined spring constant. The force acting on the cantilever is calculated via Hooke's Law as the product of its vertical displacement and spring constant. The vertical displacement is determined by monitoring the angle of reflection of a laser beam off the back of the cantilever using photodiode detectors.

In a typical AFM experiment the tip is placed in contact with the sample at a predefined repulsive force and the sample is scanned by a piezoelectric tube. During image acquisition the sample is moved up or down to ensure that the preset repulsive force is maintained. The resultant images are three-dimensional representations at constant force of sample height versus lateral probe position. This form of AFM operation is known as 'contact' mode. For reasons which become evident later, other modes of image generation have been developed which minimise tip–sample contact, i.e. the non-contact or 'tapping' modes, as also shown in Figure 4.8b and c. Tip–surface interactions can be exploited to generate data relating to the mechanical or frictional properties of material surfaces. The differential adhesion of the tip as it traverses a surface causes a distortion in the cantilever which may be translated into a lateral force or friction measurement.

There are four major reasons for the explosion in activity in AFM analysis of materials over the last decade. First, high-resolution imaging at atomic resolution for inorganic substrates and molecular resolution for organic materials is routinely accessible. Secondly, this high-resolution imaging may be undertaken in air or, much more importantly, under liquid without the need for specific sample pretreatments, such as metallic overlayers or negative staining in EM. Thirdly, the AFM is well adapted for the *in situ* examination of dynamic events such as adsorption, hydration and degradation occurring at the sample–liquid interface at molecular resolution. Finally, as the mode of operation is dependent on tip–surface interactions, the AFM can be used to explore not only topography but also local friction, compliance and even molecular interactions. In the following section each of these points is illustrated as the current and future potential of the application of AFM within biomaterials sciences.

### 4.3.2  POLYMER MORPHOLOGY

For a biomedical material, the polymer surface organisation is defined by the preparation conditions and treatments. AFM has a major role in the

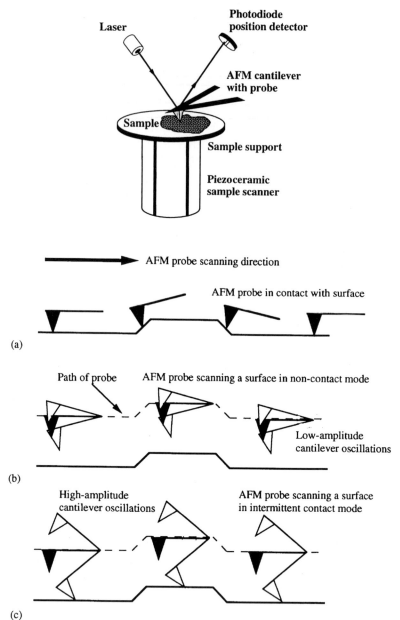

**Figure 4.8**   Schematic diagram of AFM design (a) and modes of operation (b and c)

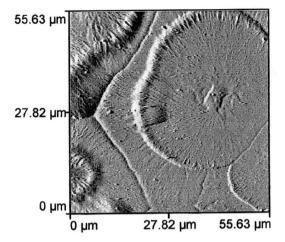

55.63 µm

27.82 µm

0 µm

0 µm          27.82 µm        55.63 µm

**Figure 4.9** AFM image (55.63×55.63 µm) of a poly(sebacic anhydride), PSA, surface revealing the presence of spherulites on the surface

characterisation of biopolymer morphology in air or under liquid. Numerous AFM studies on polymers have been reported in the literature at both high and low resolution. Molecular resolution AFM imaging (Roberts *et al.*, in press) is strictly only feasible on flat (on the nanometre scale) substrates (e.g. polymer crystals), mechanically oriented thin films, and epitaxially grown films. For example, the molecular folds in polyethylene have been imaged to determine the unit cell (Patil and Reneker, 1994). Of particular relevance to biomaterials (Sykes *et al.*, 1995) is the imaging of poly($\beta$-hydroxybutyrate), PHB, and hydroxybutyrate oligomer crystals resolving crystallographic features separated by only 0.9 nm, attributable to chain endings or folded structures.

The major application for biomaterials imaging for AFM lies in the submicrometre scale, where resolution of macromolecular assembly and organisation at the surface is the key target. A typical example of this is shown in Figure 4.9, where closely packed spherulites are clearly observed over the surface of poly(sebacic anhydride), PSA, a biodegradable polymer (Shakesheff, 1995; Shakesheff *et al.*, 1994, 1995c).

The lamella organisation (widths of *ca.* 10 nm) within the individual radiating fibres of the spherulites has been resolved for such systems. The need to characterise polymer topography is particularly necessary for complex systems, such as polymer blends, where phase separation and interfacial energetics may induce significant morphological differences. The surface morphology of PSA–PLA systems (Figure 4.10), designed for applications in drug delivery, was found to be highly influenced by blend composition, where at 50:50 composition isolated islands of PSA are dispersed within a PLA network (Shakesheff *et al.*, 1996).

Clearly such studies have implications in terms of surface engineering, where materials are blended to achieve predetermined degradation kinetics and hence

(a) 70% PSA : 30% PLA

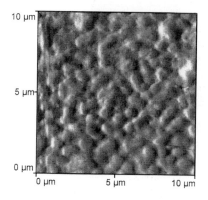

(b) 50% PSA : 50% PLA

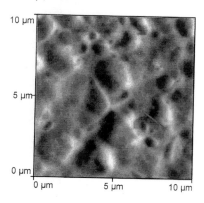

(c) 30% PSA : 70% PLA

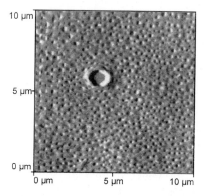

**Figure 4.10** AFM images (10 × 10 μm) of a range of PSA–PLA blends of compositions: (a) 70:30, (b) 50:50, (c) 30:70. The phase-separated domains are clearly visible on all images for these immiscible blends. At high PSA levels (70%), the PLA islands are dispersed within a PSA matrix. For the blends at the 50% and 30% PSA levels the polymers are reversed and the PSA domains are dispersed within the PLA matrix

drug release. Naturally, any form of surface treatment such as thin-film coating, plasma treatments or grafting of macromolecules designed to improve biocompatibility will have a major effect on topography, e.g. the effect of annealing of polymer latex films has provided a detailed insight into particle surface rearrangement (Goh *et al.*, 1993). AFM has a powerful role to play in the characterisation of the extent of lateral changes in interfacial structure for such processes in biomaterial development.

One area of growing interest in AFM imaging is the exploitation of lateral force in the acquisition of frictional and mechanical data to reveal surface detail not

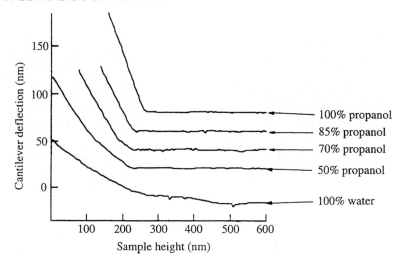

**Figure 4.11** Force curves on gelatin surfaces in propanol, water–propanol mixtures and water. The higher the water content in the mixture, the softer the gelatin surface (Radmacher *et al.*, 1995)

detectable with topographic information alone. Lateral force imaging has been able to identify the domains within surfaces of immiscible blend of poly(methyl methacrylate), PMMA, and polystyrene owing to the differences in coefficients of friction between the two materials (Motomatsu *et al.*, 1994). Of particular interest to the biomedical area is the influence of hydration of gelatin films, and this too has been studied by AFM force–displacement measurements in the dry, water and also water–propanol swollen states (Figure 4.11) (Haugstad and Gladfelter, 1994; Haugstad *et al.*, 1995b; Radmacher *et al.*, 1995). Different mechanical stiffnesses were observed for gelatin films where increasing hydration led to reduced elastic modulus of the surface, and stiffening of the interface was observed when cross-linking agents were added (Haugstad *et al.*, 1995b). Friction measurements on such surfaces suggest that the imaging process itself could be tuned by applying high tip–surface forces to induce glass–melt and glass–rubber transitions at the gelatin interface (Haugstad *et al.*, 1995a). Friction force microscopy has also been exploited to differentiate between the adsorption behaviour of fibronectin on aminosilane-covalently grafted albumin patterned arrays (Frediani *et al.*, 1994). It is interesting to note that nano-indentation AFM studies have proved much more sensitive to surface hardness of materials than the more standard micro-methods, and has therefore been exploited in producing viscoelastic images of different domains within polymer blends (Radmacher *et al.*, 1994b; Kajiyama *et al.*, 1995). Although this is a relatively new field of application, it is not difficult to envisage many exciting potential applications of tribology at biomaterial interfaces, and this sphere of activity is likely to grow rapidly.

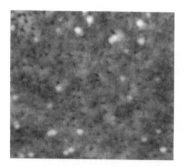 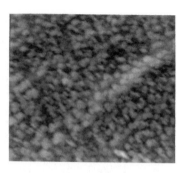

**Figure 4.12** SPM images showing the adsorption of ferritin molecules to antibody-coated ELISA well surfaces prepared either by passive adsorption or using a streptavidin–biotin protein assembly

### 4.3.3 DETERMINING BIOMOLECULAR STRUCTURE AND FUNCTION

A greater understanding of the molecular structure of biologically important molecules will contribute to our knowledge of the biochemical basis of disease and in designing chemical strategies for effective therapy. In this respect, AFM has started to make a significant contribution as a biophysical tool alongside other structural probes such as X-ray diffraction and EM (electron microscopy). The surface topography of molecules may be resolved (the inner tertiary structure is inaccessible) and gross macromolecular conformation is the key target. A number of excellent reviews exist in the literature, but one cannot really do better than the series of definitive articles on high-resolution AFM imaging of biomolecules by Shao and Yang (1995) and Shao et al. (1995, 1996).

As expected, careful attention to detail in sample preparation is crucial for reproducible high-resolution data. For molecular resolution imaging, the vast majority of the reports to date have exploited flat surfaces which have a local radius of curvature that is large in comparison to the dimensions of the AFM tip (Zasadzinski, 1996). For example, freshly cleaved mica, graphite or silicon have acted as substrates where biomolecules have been deposited using Langmuir Blodgett technology, self-assembly, electrostatic interactions, grafting via functionised surfaces and, albeit less successfully, simple deposition. Whereas the majority of AFM images within the literature have been achieved with contact mode analysis, tapping mode is growing in use, whereby possible tip-induced molecular deformation during imaging is minimised. For example, it has been shown that single globular protein molecules and protein filaments may be imaged easily and stably in buffer solution (Fritz et al., 1995). The advent of tip-deconvolution algorithms also allows a greater understanding of the influence of tip geometry on image acquisition and in determining real and artefactual features within image data (Villarrubia, 1994; Williams et al., 1996a,b). Software

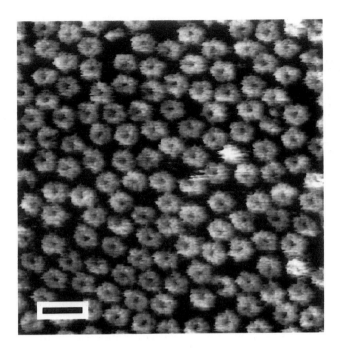

**Figure 4.13**   A high-resolution image of the cholera toxin B oligomer bound to a bilayer of egg phosphatidylcholine and the ganglioside receptor GM1. (Courtesy of Professor Shao)

algorithms have also been developed to correlate AFM data (Figure 4.12) within a molecular graphics environment (Williams *et al.*, 1991, 1994) with information available from other biophysical techniques, such as NMR and X-ray crystallography.

To date, one of the best examples of high resolution (sub-nm) imaging has been reported on the cholera toxin $\beta$ subunit oligomers randomly distributed on a phospholipid layer (Yang *et al.*, 1993). The molecule is a 85 kDa molecule with five identical subunits which bind to a ganglioside receptor placed within the supporting lipid layer (Figure 4.13). AFM images resolved the pentameric structure and the central pore of $1.8 \pm 0.2$ nm. Many other high-resolution studies have examined nucleic acid (Hansma *et al.*, 1993; Mou *et al.*, 1995), polysaccharide (Kirby *et al.*, 1995, 1996) and protein structure (Shao *et al.*, 1995, 1996). Resolving the organisation and structure within phospholipid LB films has also been a very fruitful area (Zasadzinski *et al.*, 1994; DeRose and Leblanc, 1995; Hui *et al.*, 1995). AFM has been employed to explore the molecular conformation of biomolecular interactions of importance in biology and the treatment of disease, such as protein–DNA complexes (Rees *et al.*, 1993; Erie *et al.*, 1994; Becker *et al.*, 1995; Mettikaden *et al.*, 1996; Valle *et al.*, 1996) and cytotoxic drug–DNA interactions

(Jeffrey *et al.*, 1993) respectively. Visualisation of the growth of protein crystals (Durbin *et al.*, 1993; Land *et al.*, 1995) following macromolecular assembly, e.g. amyloid filament growth associated with Alzheimer's disease (Shivji *et al.*, 1995; Stine *et al.*, 1996), observing enzyme activity (Radmacher *et al.*, 1994a) and the protein binding with membrane pore complexes (Thomson *et al.*, 1996) reflects the diverse applications and the rich vein of information available from AFM biomolecular studies.

## 4.3.4 BIOMOLECULAR–BIOMATERIAL SURFACE INTERACTIONS

### 4.3.4.1 Visualisation

There are two types of interactions between biological molecules and a material surface which are of importance in biomaterial development and performance: non-specific and specific. The former occurs on the conditioning of polymer surfaces on exposure to a biological milieu, which is the first stage in directing the host response to artificial materials. In contrast, the selective molecular recognition between a probe on a surface-engineered substrate and the complementary macromolecule in solution is exploited in a number of important biomedical devices, such as biosensors, site-specific delivery systems and chromatography. In both cases AFM can provide constructive quantitative information on the nature of the macromolecular interactions on biomaterial interfaces at molecular resolution.

The non-specific adsorption of individual molecules of a range of plasma proteins has been imaged on biomaterial interfaces at submonolayer (Cullen and Lowe, 1994; Baty *et al.*, 1996; Chen *et al.*, 1996) and also continuous films (Green *et al.*, in press).

Although valuable information may be gleaned from the nature of the monolayer formation, this approach is limited for mixed protein films as the resolution is not sufficient to resolve the protein composition, nor is it spectroscopic in nature. Despite these reservations, this area of application may have a very important role in evaluating the various interfacial modification approaches being developed within biomedical science to minimise or eradicate surface biomolecular recognition by directly visualising the reduction in protein adsorption at the nanoscale.

A high degree of selectivity and binding efficiency is a primary goal in optimising the performance of sensor devices. AFM can be employed to study microtitre well surfaces used for enzyme immunoadsorbent assays of the protein ferritin (Davies *et al.*, 1994a/b; Roberts *et al.*, 1995). By imaging the protein distribution across the polystyrene well surface, analysis was able to show that only 5% of the total antibody layer passively adsorbed on the well surface is functional, compared with 60% on biotinylated antibody bound to a streptavidin protein assembly constructed at the interface (Figure 4.14).

This AFM work has been extended to discriminate between Fab′, F(ab)$_2$, IgG and IgM molecules on such sensor substrates (Roberts *et al.*, 1995). Other studies

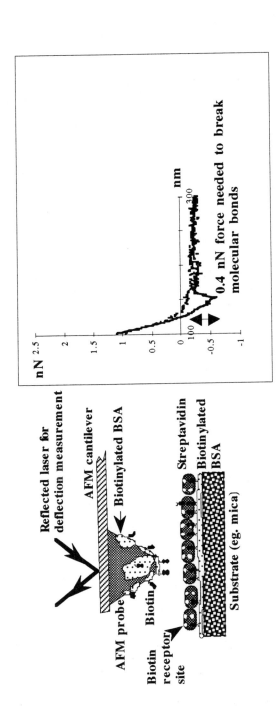

**Figure 4.14** Schematic diagram of the measurement of force–distance curves between a ligand-coated AFM tip and receptor coated on to a substrate; in this case, streptavidin and biotin

on immunocomplexes also confirm its potential as a useful sensitive screening tool (Delamarche *et al.*, 1996; Tang and McGhie, 1996). Clearly, this area of AFM study has significant implications for the development of novel immunosensors, and one can foresee that it could be readily adapted to evaluate the performance of many other biomedical devices, such as responsive delivery systems, affinity chromatographic media involved in selective dialysis of blood products, and surface modified polymer scaffolds employed in tissue engineering which are designed to elicit selective cellular interactions with surface membrane-bound biomolecular receptors.

### 4.3.4.2 Measurement

The ability of AFM to measure forces of 10 pN or less which arise from discrete intermolecular interactions has recently been highlighted (Hoh *et al.*, 1993). This work has led to a series of innovative studies which have measured the forces required to separate specific biomolecular interactions by attaching the complementary biomolecules to the AFM probe and the substrate surface (see schematic diagram in Figure 4.14). Biotin-functionalised glass beads attached to AFM cantilevers and streptavidin-coated mica surfaces have been used to estimate the strength of a single streptavidin–biotin bond (Lee *et al.*, 1994a). A similar approach was adopted to measure quantised forces of interaction between a biotinylated agarose bead and an AFM probe functionalised with avidin, a protein structurally related to streptavidin (Florin et al., 1994). This strategy has also been extended to the measurement of forces between complementary strands of DNA (Lee *et al.*, 1994b), glycoproteins (Dammer *et al.*, 1995) and antibody–antigen complexes (Hunterdorfer *et al.*, 1996), mostly on model interfaces, but the determination of interactions on industrially relevant immunoassay surfaces has recently been reported (Allen *et al.*, 1996). In this respect, AFM is being accepted as a major biophysical tool for the evaluation of discrete molecular forces. In another twist on the AFM measurement of surface interactions, force–distance AFM studies on PEO-grafted surfaces revealed significant repulsion between tip and surface owing to the PEO steric layer (Lea *et al.*, 1994) and suggests a future role for this approach in evaluating protein-resistant polymer brushes grafted on to biomaterials.

This work has been extended where a force microscope has been used to measure the adhesive and friction forces between functional group modified tips and organic surfaces with defined functionalities (Frisbie *et al.*, 1994; Noy *et al.*, 1995). The adhesive interactions between the functionalities, i.e. $CH_3:CH_3$, $CH_3:COOH$ and $COOH:COOH$, were shown to correlate directly with friction images of the surfaces patterned with functional groups. Mapping the spatial arrangements of functional groups on such surfaces has significant implications in defining medical materials and biological systems. An exciting projection of this approach to mapping with biomolecule-grafted tips may permit the localisation of antigens or specific recognition sites on cells or biosensor arrays.

(a)                                          (b)

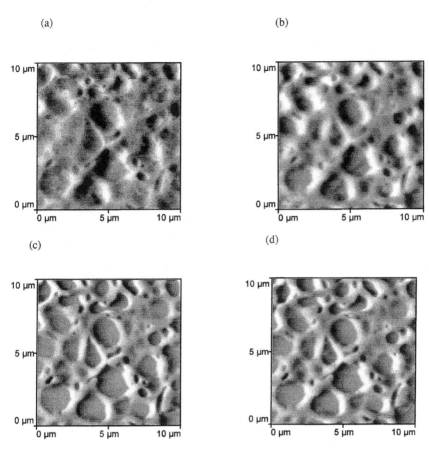

(c)                                          (d)

**Figure 4.15** AFM images (10 × 10 μm) of the degradation of PSA–PLA blend (50:50 composition) at pH 12.5 after 0, 5, 10 and 20 minutes. The loss of the rapidly degrading PSA islands leaves a slower-degrading PLA network. (a) 0 min; (b) 5 min; (c) 10 min; (d) 20 min

### 4.3.4.3 Dynamic Studies

The ability to image surfaces within an aqueous environment has being exploited in a number of AFM studies on biomaterials examining dynamic processes such as erosion, hydration and adsorption at interfaces.

Biodegradable polymers are being exploited for a wide range of biomedical applications and there is considerable interest in the nature of the degradation mechanism. The morphology of such material will influence the erosion process, where crystalline regions will inhibit water ingress, resulting in preferential degradation of amorphous regions where water diffusion is preferred. This phenomenon has been observed in the rapid degradation and loss of amorphous material during the AFM imaging of melt-crystallised PSA films in buffer,

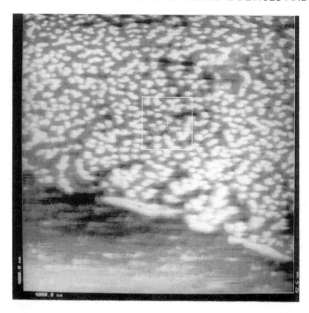

**Figure 4.16**   AFM images (4 × 4 μm) of a submonolayer of albumin molecules at a polystyrene surface

resulting in the exposure of crystalline fibres that are less susceptible to degradation (Shakesheff *et al.*, 1994, 1995c). Polymer blend composition may also have a significant impact on the degradation kinetics. AFM studies, as shown in Figure 4.15, have revealed differential degradation rates for blends of PSA–PLA, so demonstrating the rapid erosion of the PSA component of the surface, while the porous PLA network remains intact (Shakesheff *et al.*, 1996).

This work has been extended to visualise in real time the simultaneous erosion of a degradable poly(orthoester) system and the release of a model protein, bovine serum albumin (BSA), dispersed within the polymer matrix (Shakesheff *et al.*, 1995a).

It has been noted that the hydration of a biomaterial is likely to result in the considerable restructuring of the interfacial chemistry, and this naturally will have a profound effect on the surface morphology and, as shown for gelatin, the surface mechanical properties. AFM has also been employed to monitor changes in the electroactive polymers where changes in sample height allowed the swelling of the polymer to be followed (Nyffenegger *et al.*, 1995). The structural reorganisation of perfluorinated membrane polymers has also been studied in a similar manner (Chomakova-Haefke *et al.*, 1994); it is postulated that the disordered network structure of the dry state is transformed on swelling to an ordered structure of parallel fibrils. It is evident that such a strategy may be extremely valuable for the more widespread nanoscale study of biomaterial interfaces where hydration is a key requirement for performance, e.g. thin-film technology, responsive delivery systems and hydrogels.

The conditioning of biomaterial surfaces is a key stage in determining the biocompatibility of medical implants and in the development of novel delivery systems, biosensors and immunoassays. To date, there have been just a few studies which have shown that AFM can provide *in situ* dynamic data on the local nature of protein adsorption processes (Figure 4.16).

The influence of time and concentration on the development of a monolayer of fibrinogen molecules on polystyrene surfaces has been studied in buffer at molecular resolution using AFM (Chen *et al.*, 1996). Other studies have investigated the effect of protein nucleation and spreading in the generation of monolayers of fibrinogen and glucose oxidase (Cullen and Lowe, 1994). Interestingly, the AFM data suggested that the glucose oxidase was denatured by the adsorption process. Although this approach is limited in that it is unable to identify the protein composition of monolayers generated from complex biological fluids such as serum, plasma or urine, the visualisation of the formation of these layers is important in understanding the initial events in the kinetics, growth and lateral arrangement of these protein films.

### 4.3.5   FUTURE DIRECTIONS

It is clear from the previous sections that there is a considerable range of potential applications for AFM instruments in the study of biomaterials and the biomedical sciences from fundamental studies of macromolecular interactions to the development of advanced medical devices. It is evident that the field is not static: there are rapid advances in instrumentation, including the development of a cryogenic AFM for the radically improved high-resolution imaging of biomolecular structure (Han *et al.*, 1995). The advent of this technology has also led to a range of new microscopies, which are variants on its construction and are designed to measure discrete surface properties, e.g. scanning near-field optical microscopes (SNOM) employ a fibreoptic tip which has allowed the near-molecular resolution imaging of fluorescently labelled molecules at surfaces (Rucker *et al.*, 1995). The scanning thermal (Song *et al.*, 1995), electric force (Viswanathan and Heaney, 1995) and magnetic force microscopes (Proksch *et al.*, in press) are among a suite of new instruments which have been constructed in the last decade. AFMs have also been combined with other instrumentation, including light microscopy, EM and surface plasmon resonance, SPR (Chen *et al.*, 1995; Shakesheff *et al.*, 1995b). Many of these new technologies have considerable potential for the study of biomedical systems.

## 4.4   ADDITIONAL COMPLEMENTARY SURFACE TECHNIQUES

There are a number of additional surface methodologies which offer valuable data in the characterisation of specific physicochemical properties of biomaterial surfaces.

Fourier Transform infrared, FT-IR, (Andrade, 1985b) is a very useful surface spectroscopy. Although the sampling depth of this technique at best renders the data of near-surface (1 $\mu$m) quality, important information has been derived for a number of systems. FT-IR is able to provide valuable information on the molecular structure, conformation, orientation, inter- and intramolecular interactions of materials, and a number of elegant studies have shown that FT-IR may be employed to quantify the adsorption of proteins (Giroux and Cooper, 1991) and potentially probe the conformation of biomolecules at interfaces. There are a number of important approaches which allow the dynamic *in situ* study of biomaterial–biomolecule interactions. SPR has only very recently been applied to the study of biomaterial systems (Davies *et al.*, 1992). SPR is an evanescent wave technique which monitors the refractive index above a noble metal sensor, with a maximum sampling depth of 100 nm above the surface. SPR is able to monitor dynamic kinetic surface processes such as adsorption phenomena, degradation or hydration by sensing the change in the dielectric properties at the interface. The sensitivity of instrumentation has been quoted at around $10^{-16}$ mol mm$^{-2}$ for a 150 kDa protein. Commercial SPR instruments are now available which allow the analysis of the kinetics and affinity constants for receptor–ligand interactions which are making a major impact in molecular biology (Karlsson *et al.*, 1991; Fagerstam *et al.*, 1992). In biomaterials development the technique has proved very valuable for studying protein adsorption on self-assembly monolayers (Prime and Whitesides, 1993) and macromolecular assemblies (Davies *et al.*, 1994b). By coating the metal substrate with a thin film of the biomedical polymer of interest, protein adsorption may be followed directly in real time (Van Delden *et al.*, in press) and changes in polymer structure such as degradation (Chen *et al.*, 1995; Shakesheff *et al.*, 1995b; Chen *et al.*, 1996) and hydration (Green, unpublished results) may be monitored. The dynamic *in situ* nature of the information, allowing valuable kinetic data to be derived from surface processes, suggests SPR should have a valuable impact in biomaterial characterisation. Ellipsometry (Davies *et al.*, 1992) is more established in this area of the biomedical sciences and has been employed in a number of surface studies in the literature, in dynamic measurements of the thickness and refractive index of adsorbed protein layers (Greef, 1990; Horbett and Brash, 1995) and dynamic changes in film structure.

The use of contact angle data of liquids on surfaces in defining the wettability and surface energetics of biomaterials is a common feature of many biomaterial studies (Andrade, 1985a). A number of approaches have been developed for contact angle measurement, from the sessile drop to the Wilhelmy plate technique (Andrade, 1985a). A number of theoretical models exist for the derivation of material surface energies in terms of polar and dispersion forces. The Wilhelmy plate technique is particularly useful for time-dependent studies which follow dynamic surface changes. Dynamic contact angle analysis (by dipping the polymer-coated plate into and out of a liquid in a controlled manner) also allows the continuous measurement of data over the entire surface and, from the differential between the advancing and receding angles, important information may be determined on changes in surface structure. The reorientation of surface groups and swelling and hydration of interfacial layers have also been followed using this approach (Andrade, 1985a). As the contact data are derived from the top molecular layer of the surface, it is very sensitive to the study of adsorption phenomena such as protein conditioning (Davies *et al.*, 1992). Dynamic contact angle measurements were found to be more sensitive to albumin adsorption on to silicone tubing than ToF–SIMS (Davies *et al.*, 1996). Naturally, contact angle measurements are a very powerful tool for the measurement of the degree of changes in wettability after the interfacial modification of biomaterial interfaces.

## 4.5  CONCLUSION

This chapter has presented (from a personal viewpoint) the key methodologies for defining the interfacial chemistry of biomaterials. The dynamic and complex environment of these systems, which is extremely challenging to define and characterise, has been noted. The chapter has reaffirmed that no one technique has the necessary range to describe all the properties of an interface, and that the most fruitful conclusions are drawn from a comprehensive surface analysis of a biomaterial system which is directly correlated to appropriate biological indicators. With time, our increasing depth of knowledge of biomedical colloid and surface chemistry is illustrating how little we really know about the biointeractions occurring at material surfaces. As key questions on surface phenomena come to the fore, we as a community need to devise new analytical approaches to probe each issue. This has been a strong feature of surface analysis of biomaterials over the last decade, but this area of innovation needs to be maintained. As increasing pressures fall on industry to ensure the quality and efficacy of biomedical materials and devices, and with the advent of second-generation biomaterials with well-defined and engineered properties for advanced medical and therapeutic applications, there can be no doubt that surface analysis techniques can play a significant role in developing our understanding of the physicochemical properties of conventional and advanced biomedical systems and make a valuable contribution in interpreting their biological performance.

## 4.6  REFERENCES

Absolom DR, Zing W, van Oss CJ and Neumann AW (1984) Biomat Med Dev Art Org 12:235.
Alexander MR, Wright PV and Ratner BD (1996) Surf Interf Anal 24(3):217–220.
Allen S, Davies J, Dawkes AC *et al.* (1996) Febs Lett 390:161.
Andrade JD (ed.) (1985a) Surface and interfacial aspects of biomedical polymers 1: Surface chemistry and physics. Plenum Press, New York, USA.

Andrade JD (ed.) (1985b) Surface and interfacial aspects of biomedical polymers 2: Protein adsorption. Plenum Press, New York, USA.

Batts GN and Paul AJ (1994) Langmuir 10(1):218.

Baty AM, Suci PA, Tyler BJ and Geesey GG (1996) J Coll Interf Sci 177(2):307.

Beamson G and Briggs D (1992) High resolution XPS of organic polymers: The Scienta ESCA300 database. Wiley, Chichester, UK.

Becker JC, Nikroo A, Brabletz T and Reisfeld RA (1995) Proc Natl Acad Sci USA 92(21):9727.

Benninghoven A and Rading D (1994) Macromol Symp 83:27.

Binnig G (1992) Ultramicroscopy 42-44A:7–15.

Blestos IV, Hercules DM, Greifendorf D and Benninghoven A (1985) Anal Chem 57:2384.

Bridgett J, Davies MC, Denyer SP and Watts JF. Biomaterials, in press.

Briggs D and Hearn MJ (1985) Int J Mass Spectrom – Ion Processes 67:47.

Briggs D and Munro HS (1987) Polym Comm 28:307.

Briggs D and Ratner BD (1988) Polym Comm 29:6.

Briggs D and Seah MP (eds) (1990) Practical surface analysis 1: Auger and X-ray photoelectron spectroscopy. Wiley, Chichester, UK.

Briggs D and Seah MP (eds) (1992) Practical surface analysis 2: Ion and neutral spectroscopy. Wiley, Chichester, UK.

Briggs D, Hearn MJ and Ratner BD (1984) Surf Interf Anal 6:184.

Brindley A, Davis SS, Davies MC and Watts JF (1995) J Coll Interf Sci 171:150.

Brinkhaus PH and van Ooij WJ (1988) Surf Interf Anal 11:214.

Brown A and Vickerman JC (1986) Surf Interf Anal 8:75.

Bruil A, Brenneisen LM, Terlingen JGA et al. (1994) J Coll Interf Sci 165(1):72.

Burnham NA and Colton RJ (1993) In: Scanning tunnelling microscopy and spectroscopy: theory, techniques and applications. Bonnell DA (ed). VCH, New York, USA.

Callen BW, Sodhi RNS, Shelton RM and Davies JE (1993) J Biomed Mater Res 27(7):851.

Castner DG, Lewis KB, Fischer DA, Ratner BD and Gland JL (1993) Langmuir 9(2):537.

Chen X, Shakesheff KM, Davies MC et al. (1995) J Phys Chem 99:11537.

Chen X, Davies MC, Roberts CJ et al. (1996) Anal Chem 68:1451.

Chilkoti A and Ratner BD (1993) In: Surface characterisation of advanced polymers. Sabbatini L and Zambonin PG (eds). VCH, Weinheim.

Chilkoti A, Ratner BD and Briggs D (1993a) Anal Chem 65(13):1736.

Chilkoti A, Lopez GP, Ratner BD, Hearn MJ and Briggs D (1993b) Macromol 26(18):4825.

Chomakova-Haefke M, Nyffenegger R and Schmidt E (1994) Appl Phys A 59:151.

Cullen DC and Lowe CR (1994) J Coll Interf Sci 166:102.

Dammer U, Popescu O, Wagner P et al. (1995) Science 267:1173.

Davies J, Allen A, Bruce I et al. (1992) In: Proceedings of Intl Conf on surface properties of biomaterials. Batts G and West RH (eds). Butterworth Heinemann, Oxford.

Davies J, Dawkes AC, Haymes AG et al. (1994a) J Immunol Meth 167:263.

Davies J, Roberts CJ, Dawkes AC et al. (1994b) Langmuir 110:2654.

Davies J, Nunnerley CS and Paul AJ (1996) Coll Surf Biointeract 6:181.

Davies MC and Brown A (1987) In: Controlled release technology: pharmaceutical applications. ACS Symp Ser 348, Washington DC, USA.

Davies MC, Short RD, Newton JM and Chapman SR (1988a) Surf Interf Anal 11:591.

Davies MC, Khan MA, Brown A and Humphrey P (1988b) In: SIMS VI. Benninghoven A, Huber AM and Werner HW (eds). Wiley, Chichester, UK.

Davies MC, Short RD, Khan MA et al. (1989) Surf Interf Anal 14:115.

Davies MC and Lynn RAP (1990) Crit Rev Biocompat 5(40):297.

Davies MC, Lynn RAP, Watts JF et al. (1991) Macromol 24:5508.

Davies MC, Lynn RAP, Davis SS et al. (1993a) J Coll Interf Sci 156:229.

Davies MC, Lynn RAP, Davis SS et al. (1993b) Langmuir 9(7):1637.

Davies MC, Lynn RAP, Davis SS et al. (1994) Langmuir 10:1399.

Davies MC, Lynn RAP, Hearn MJ et al. (1996) Langmuir 12:3866.
Davis SS, Illum L, Moghimi SM et al. (1993) J Contr Release 24:157.
Delamarche E, Sundarababu G, Biebuyck H et al. (1996) Langmuir 12(8):1997.
De Rose JA and Leblanc RM (1995) Surf Sci Rep 22:73.
Dewez JL, Schneider YL and Rouxhet PG (1996) J Biomed Mater Res 30(3):373.
Dombrowski KE, Wright SE, Birbeck JC and Moddeman WE (1996) FASEB J 10(6):2854.
Dunn SE, Brindley A, Davis SS, Davies MC and Illum L (1994) Pharm Res 11(7):1456.
Durbin SD, Carlson WE and Saros MT (1993) J Phys D – Appl Phys 26:B128.
Elwing H, Welin S, Askendal A, Nilsson U and Lundstrom I (1987) J Coll Interf Sci 119:203.
Erie DA, Yang G, Schultz HC and Bustamante C (1994) Science 266:1562.
Fagerstam LG, Frostell-Karlsson A, Karlsson R, Persson B and Ronnberg I (1992) J Chromatogr 597:397.
Fakes DW, Davies MC, Brown A and Newton JM (1988) Surf Interf Anal 13:233.
Feast WJ and Munro HS (eds)(1987) Polymer surfaces and interfaces. Wiley, Chichester, UK.
Feast WJ, Munro HS and Richards RW (eds) (1993) Polymer surfaces and interfaces II. Wiley, Chichester, UK.
Ferruti P, Barbucci R, Danzo N et al. (1982) Biomaterials 3:33.
Florin E-L, Moy VT and Gaub HE (1994) Science 264:415.
France RM, OToole L, Short RD and Pollicino N (1995) Macromol Chem Phys 196(11):3695.
Frediani C, Allegrini M, Ascoli C et al. (1994) Nanotechnol 5:95.
Frisbie C, Daniel F, Rozsnyai F, Noy A and Wrighton MS (1994) Science 265:2071.
Fritz M, Radmacker M, Cleveland JP et al. (1995) Langmuir 11:3529.
Garbassi F and Carli F (1986) Surf Interf Anal 8:229.
Gilding DK, Paynter RW and Castle JE (1990) Biomaterials 1:163.
Giroux TA and Cooper SL (1991) J Coll Interf Sci 146:179.
Goh MC, Juhue D, Leung OM, Wang Y and Winnik MA (1993) Langmuir 9:1319.
Greef R (1990) In: Surface analysis techniques and applications. Randell DR and Neagle W (eds). RSC, Cambridge, UK.
Green RJ, Davies J, Davies MC, Roberts CJ and Tendler SJB. Biomaterials, in press.
Griffith A, Glidle A and Cooper JM (1996) Biosens Bioelectron 11(6-7):625.
Hagenhoff B (1995) Biosens Bioelectron 10(9-10):885.
Han W, Mou J, Sheng J, Yang J and Shao ZF (1995) Biochem 34:8215.
Hansma HG, Sinsheimer RL, Groppe J et al. (1993) Scanning 15(5):296.
Hansma PK, Cleveland JP Radmacher M et al. (1994) Appl Phys Lett 64:1738.
Hanson SR, Harker LA, Ratner BD and Hoffman AS (1982) In: Biomaterials 1980: Advances in biomaterials 3. Winter GD, Gibbons GF and Plenk H (eds). Wiley, Chichester, UK.
Haugstad G and Gladfelter WL (1994) Ultramicroscopy 54:31.
Haugstad G, Gladfelter WL, Weberg EB, Weberg RT and Jones RR (1995a) Langmuir 11:3473.
Haugstad G, Gladfelter WG, Weberg EB (1995b) Mat Sci Eng C – Biomimetic Mat Sens Syst 3(2):85.
Hearn MJ, Briggs D, Yoon SC and Ratner BD (1987) Surf Interf Anal 10:384.
Hearn MJ, Ratner BD and Briggs D (1988) Macromol 21:2950.
Hoh JH, Cleveland JP, Pratter CB, Revel J-P and Hansma PK (1993) J Am Chem Soc 114:4917.
Horbett TA and Brash JL (1995) Proteins at interfaces II: Fundamentals and applications. ACS Symp Ser 602, Washington DC, USA.
Hui SW, Viswanathan R, Zasadzinski JA and Israelachvili JN (1995) Biophys J 68:171.
Hunterdorfer P, Baumgartner W, Gruber HJ, Schilcher K and Schindler H (1996) Proc Nat Acad Sci 93:3477.
Illum L and Davis SS (1987) Life Sci 40:1553.

Jeffrey AM, Jing TW, DeRose JA et al. (1993) Nucl Acid Res 21:5896.
John CM, Odom RW, Salvati I, Annapragada A and Lu MYF (1995) Anal Chem 67:21.
Kajiyama T, Ohki I, Tanaka K, Ge SR and Takahara A (1995) Proc Jpn Acad B – Phys and Biol Sci 2:75.
Karlsson R, Michaelson A and Mattsson L (1991) J Immunol Meth 145:229.
Kirby AR, Gunning AP and Morris VJ (1995) Carbohydr Res 267:161.
Kirby AR, Gunning AP and Morris VJ (1996) Biopolymers 38:355.
Klee D, Severich B and Hocker H (1996) Macromol Symp 103:19-29.
Koosha F, Muller RH, Davis SS and Davies MC (1989) J Contr Release 9:149.
Land TA, Malkin AJ, Kuznetsov YG, McPherson A and Deyoreo JJ (1995) Phys Rev Lett 75(14):2774.
Lea AS, Andrade JD and Hlady V (1994) Colloid Surf A – Physicochem Eng Aspects 93:349.
Lee GU, Kidwell DA and Colton RJ (1994a) Langmuir 10:354.
Lee GU, Chrisey LA and Colton RJ (1994b) Science 266:771.
Lee S-D, Hsiue G-H, Kao C-Y and Chang PC-T (1996) Biomaterials 17:587.
Leggett G and Downes S. Langmuir, in press.
Leggett GJ, Briggs D and Vickerman JC (1990a) J Chem Soc – Farad Trans 86:1863.
Leggett GJ, Briggs D and Vickerman JC (1990b) Surf Interf Anal 16:3.
Leggett GL, Vickerman JC, Briggs D and Hearn MJ (1992) J Chem Soc – Farad Trans 88:297.
Leggett GJ, Davies MC, Roberts CJ et al. (1993) Langmuir 9:2356.
Leggett GJ, Ratner BD and Vickerman JC (1995) Surf Interf Anal 23(1):22.
Leute A, Rading D, Benninghoven A, Schroeder K and Klee D (1994) Adv Mater 6(10):775-780.
Lewis KB and Ratner BD (1993) J Coll Interf Sci 158:77.
Lhoest JB, Dewez JL and Bertrand P (1995a) Nucl Instr Meth Phys Res B – Beam interactions with materials and atoms 105(1-4):322.
Lhoest JB, Bertrand P, Weng LT and Dewez JL (1995b) Macromol 28(13):4631.
Lin HB, Lewis KB, Leachscampavia D, Ratner BD and Cooper SL (1993) J Biomed Sci – Polym Ed 4(3):183.
Linton RW, Desimone JM, Beli AM et al. (1996) ACS 211(2):337.
Lopez GP, Ratner BD, Raposa RJ and Horbett TA (1993) Macromol 26(13):3247.
Lub J, van Vroonhoven FCBM, van Leyen D and Benninghoven A (1987) J Polym Sci – Polym Phys Ed 27:2071.
Lub J and van Velzen PNT (1989) In: Ion formation from organic solids (IFOSS), VI. Benninghoven A (ed.). Wiley, Chichester, UK.
Magnani A, Barbucci R, Lewis KB, Leachscampavia D and Ratner BD (1995) J Mat Chem 5(9):1321.
Mantus DS, Ratner BD, Carlson BA and Moulder JF (1993) Anal Chem 65(10):1431.
Marti O and Amrein M (eds) (1993) STM & SFM in biology. Academic Press, California, USA.
McLafferty FW and Turecek F (1993) Interpretation of mass spectrometry, 4th edn. University Science Books, Mill Valley, California, USA.
Mettikadan S, Yu H, Tokumasu F, Kolattukudy P and Takeyasu K (1996) Biophys J 70(2):462.
Missirlis YF and Lemm W (1991) Modern aspects of protein adsorption on biomaterials. Kluwer Academic Publishers, Dordrecht, The Netherlands.
Motomatsu M, Nie H-Y, Mizutani W and Tokumoto H (1994) Jpn J Appl Phys 33:3375.
Mou JX, Czajkowsky DM, Zhang YY and Shao ZF (1995) Febs Lett 371:279.
Mrksich M, Segal GB and Whitesides GM (1995) Langmuir 11:4383.
Muddiman DC, Nicola AJ, Proctor A and Hercules DM (1996) Appl Spectrosc 50(2):161.
Noy A, Frisbie CD, Rozsnyai LF, Wrighton MS and Lieber CM (1995) J Am Chem Soc 117:7943.

Nyffenegger R, Ammann E, Siegenthaler H, Kotz R and Hass O (1995) Electrochemica Acta 40:1411.

Overney RH, Meyer E, Frommer J et al. (1992) Nature 359:133.

Park D, Keszler B, Galiatsatos V, Kennedy JP and Ratner BD (1995) Macromol 28(8): 2595.

Park A and Cima LG (1996) J Biomed Mater Res 31(1):117.

Patil R and Reneker DH (1994) Polymer 35:1909.

Patrick JS, Cooks RG and Pachuta SJ (1994) Biolog Mass Spectrom 23(11):653.

Perezluna VH, Horbett TA and Ratner BD (1994) J Biomed Mater Res 28(10):1111.

Petrat FM, Wolany D, Schwede BC, Wiedman L and Benninghoven A (1994a) Surf Interf Anal 21(5):274.

Petrat FM, Wolany D, Schwede BC, Wiedman L and Benninghoven A (1994b) Surf Interf Anal 21(5):402.

Prime KL and Whitesides GM (1993) JACS 115:10714.

Proksch R, Runge E and Hansma PK. J Appl Phys, in press.

Quate CF (1994) Surf Sci 299-300:980.

Radmacher M, Fritz M, Hansma HG and Hansma PK (1994a) Science 265:1577.

Radmacher M, Fritz M, Cleveland JP, Waters DA and Hansma PK (1994b) Langmuir 10:3809.

Radmacher M, Fritz M and Hansma PK (1995) Biophys J 69:264.

Ratner BD (ed.) (1988) Surface characterisation of biomaterials. Prog in Biomed Eng 6, Elsevier Science, Amsterdam, The Netherlands.

Ratner BD (1993) Cardiovasc Cardiol 2(3):S87.

Ratner BD, Leachscampavia D and Castner DG (1993) Biomaterials 14(2):148.

Ratner BD (1995) Surf Interf Anal 23:521.

Reichlmaier S, Hammond JS, Hearn MJ and Briggs D (1994) Surf Interf Anal 21(11):739.

Reichlmaier S, Bryan SR and Briggs D (1995) J Vac Sci Technol A – Vac Surf Films 13(3):1217.

Rees WA, Keller RW, Vesenka JP, Yang G and Bustamante C (1993) Science 260:1646.

Riviere JC (ed.) (1990) Surface analytical techniques. Clarendon Press, Oxford, UK.

Roberts CJ, Williams PM, Davies J et al. (1995) Langmuir 11:1822.

Roberts CJ, Davies MC, Shakesheff KM, Tendler SJB and Williams PM. Trends Polym Sci. in press.

Ruardy TG, Schakenraad JM, van der Mei HC and Busscher HJ (1995) J Biomed Mater Res 29:1415.

Rucker M, Vanoppen P, de Schryver FC, ter Host JJ, Hotta J and Masuhara H (1995) Macromol 28:7530.

Sabbatini L and Zambonin PG (eds) (1993) Surface characterisation of advanced polymers. VCH, Weinheim, Germany.

Schakenra JM, Busscher HJ, Wildevuur ChR and Arends J (1984). J Biomed Mater Res 20:773.

Shakesheff KM (1995) PhD Thesis, University of Nottingham, UK.

Shakesheff KM, Davies MC, Domb A et al. (1994) Langmuir 10:4417.

Shakesheff KM, Davies MC, Heller J et al. (1995a) Langmuir 11:2547.

Shakesheff KM, Chen X, Davies MC et al. (1995b) Langmuir 11:3921.

Shakesheff KM, Davies MC, Domb A et al. (1995c) Macromol 28:1108.

Shakesheff KM, Davies MC, Shard AG et al. (1996) Macromol 29:2205.

Shao ZF and Yang J (1995) Quart Rev Biophys 28(2):195.

Shao ZF, Yang J and Somlyo AP (1995) Ann Rev Cell Dev Biol 11:241.

Shao ZF, Mou J, Czajkowsky DM, Yang J and Yuan JY (1996) Adv Phys 45(1):1.

Shard AG, Davies MC, Tendler SJB et al. (1995) Polymer 36(4):775.

Shard AG, Volland C, Davies MC and Kissel T (1996) Macromol 29:748.

Shard AG, Schacht E and Davies MC. Surf Interf Anal, in press.

Sheu MS, Hoffman AS, Ratner BD, Feijen J and Harris JM (1993) J Adhes Sci Technol 7(10):1065.
Shivji AP, Davies MC, Roberts CJ, Tendler SJB and Wilkinson MJ Prot Peptide Lett.
Song M, Hammiche A, Pollock HM, Hourston DJ and Reading MS (1995) Polymer 36:3313.
Steele JG (1995) ACS Symp Series 602:436.
Steffens P, Niehuis E, Freise T, Greifendorf D and Benninghoven A (1985) J Vac Sci Technol A3:1322.
Stenger DA, Pike CJ, Hickman JJ and Cotman CW (1993) Brain Res 630(1-2):136.
Stine WB, Synder SW, Ladror US et al. (1996) J Prot Chem 15(2):193.
Subirade M and Lebugle A (1994) Thin Solid Films 243(1-2):442.
Sugiyama K, Shiraishi K, Ohga K et al. (1993) Polym J 25(5):512.
Sugiyama K and Oku T (1995) Polym J 27(2):179.
Swalen JD (1987) Langmuir 3:932.
Sykes KE, McMaster TJ, Miles MJ et al. (1995) J Mat Sci 30:623.
Tang SL and McGhie AJ (1996) Langmuir 12(4):1088.
Thomson NH, Fritz M, Radmacher M et al. (1996) Biophys J 70(5):2421.
Tyler BJ, Castner DG and Ratner BD (1989) Surf Interf Anal 14:443.
Valle M, Valpuesta JM, Carrascosa JL, Tamayo J and Garcia R (1996) J Struct Biol 116(3):390.
Van Delden CJ, Lens JP, Kooyman RPH, Engbers GHM and Feijen J. Biomaterials, in press.
Vickerman JC and Briggs D (eds) (1996) The Wiley static SIMS library. Wiley, Chichester, UK.
Villarrubia J (1994) Surf Sci 321:287.
Viswanathan R and Heaney MB (1995) Phys Rev Lett 75:4433.
Walls JM (ed.) (1990) Methods of surface analysis: techniques and applications. Cambridge University Press, Cambridge, UK.
Ward AJ and Short RD (1995) Polymer 36(18):3439.
Weng LT, Betrand P, Stone-Masui JH and Stone WEE (1994) Surf Interf Anal 21:87.
Weng LT, Bertrand P, Lauer W, Zimmer R and Busetti S (1995) Surf Interf Anal 23:879.
Wilcox MH (1993) In: Microbial biofilms: formation and control. Denyer SP, Gorman SP and Sussman M (eds). Blackwell Scientific, Oxford, UK.
Williams PM, Davies MC, Jackson DE et al. (1991) Nanotechol 2:172.
Williams PM, Davies MC, Jackson DE, Roberts CJ and Tendler SJB (1994) J Vac Sci Technol B 12:1517.
Williams PM, Shakesheff KM, Davies MC et al. (1996a) J Vac Sci Technol B 14:1432.
Williams PM, Davies MC, Jackson DE et al. (1996b) Langmuir 12:3468.
Yang J, Tamm LKI, Toillack TW and Shao ZF (1993) J Mol Biol 229:286.
Yoon SC, Ratner BD, Ivan B and Kennedy JP (1994) Macromol 27(6):548.
Zasadzinski JA, Viswanathan R, Shwartz DK et al. (1994) Coll Surf A 93:305.
Zasadzinski JA (1996) Curr Opin Coll Interf Sci 1:264.
Zhuang H and Gardella JA (1996) MRS Bulletin Jan:43.
Zimmerman PA and Hercules DM (1994) Appl Spectrosc 48(5):620-622.

# 5

# Sterilisation Processes and Residuals

VICTOR DORMAN-SMITH
Abbott Ireland, Sligo, Ireland

## 5.1 INTRODUCTION

It may be wondered what the link is between the issues relevant to sterilisation and those concerning biocompatibility. The simple answer is that most medical devices, for which biocompatibility is an important factor, are normally sterile at the time of use, in particular implants, other invasive devices and those in contact with breached skin.

This chapter only addresses the generalities of sterilisation and its effect on the evaluation of biocompatibility. It is not intended to be an in-depth discussion on all aspects of device sterilisation, but an introduction to the subject indicating those related aspects which are most important in supplying safe medical devices. For those requiring greater detail the recent book by Morrisey and Briggs-Phillips (1993) is recommended.

When assessing the biocompatibility of 'finished' (i.e. ready to use) devices, it is most important to carry out tests on the sterilised device. In that way, any differences between the raw materials used in the manufacture of the device and the same material after transformation (e.g. moulding, grinding, welding, coating etc.) and including the effects of any sterilisation procedure used (e.g. residues, degradation, heat etc.), can be determined.

It is normal practice when designing a device that will be provided sterile, to consider the effect of the proposed sterilisation procedure on the materials used. Typical effects will be discussed later. The sterilisation procedure may also have an effect on the sterile package integrity and/or on the functionality of the device. These should also be addressed, both at the design stage and during validation of the product.

Sterilisation is an example of a process whose efficacy cannot be verified by inspection or non-destructive testing. What is 'sterile'? 'Sterile' is normally defined in absolute terms as 'the condition of a medical device that is free from

*Biocompatibility Assessment of Medical Devices and Materials.*
Edited by Julian Braybrook. © 1997 John Wiley & Sons Ltd.

**Figure 5.1**   Symbol No. 1051 for 'single-use device'

viable microorganisms' (EN 556), but this is not very helpful when evaluating for sterility since the absence of 'something' is practically impossible to prove. The purpose of all sterilisation processes is to inactivate any microbiological contaminants that may be present on the device. In practice, this is found to approximate to an exponential curve, so that knowledge of the initial bacterial load and the rate of kill of the process leads to a statistical estimate of the possible non-sterility of any one item in a batch of sterilised product. Hence it has become standard practice to specify sterility in terms of a risk of non-sterility. This risk may be defined in standards (e.g. EN 556) or may be subject to regulatory agreement, and may vary with varying product end-use. In any case, the sterilisation procedure must be part of the specification for a sterile product.

Many sterile devices are designed and supplied to be used once and then discarded – so-called 'single-use' devices. A symbol that is becoming more familiar these days in hospitals is number 1051 in ISO 7000 (Figure 5.1).

Although this is not the place for a discussion on 'single-use' versus 'reusable' devices, it is enough to note that devices supplied sterile and designated as 'single use' by the manufacturer have been made from approved materials in a controlled environment and have been subjected to a qualified sterilisation process. Any attempt to reuse them by cleaning followed by resterilising is fraught with so many pitfalls that it is doubtful whether anyone can guarantee that the devices will have the same specification and performance as they had originally.

In recent years, especially since the harmonised 'new approach' Directives in the European Union (EU) covering medical devices, and the reliance of those Directives on standards, a number of standards have been written at European and ISO levels covering both sterilisation processes and associated requirements, such as biological indicators, packaging, the measurement of bioburden and sterilisation residues. These are covered later in this chapter. In addition, because many pharmaceuticals are required to be sterile, the Pharmacopoeias have contained monographs on sterilisation processes for some time, but these have tended to be general and informative in nature.

As already indicated in Chapter 1, standards are generally written to be voluntary, but if a sterilisation process standard is to be useful it needs to detail conditions that can guarantee the sterility of the products subject to the process. It may, however, also include guidance on how the 'requirements' in the standard can be fulfilled. In the case of the EU medical device Directives, the European standards play a special role if they are 'harmonised' (in the sense of being listed in the European *Official Journal*). They can be used by the manufacturer in the knowledge that the third-party assessor (the Notified Body) must accept the standard as complying with the essential requirements of the Directive. It follows, therefore, that some standards are taking on the role of *de facto* regulations.

Facilities and equipment for carrying out sterilisation can be very expensive, so many small manufacturers have opted to sterilise their devices at a specialist contract steriliser and thereby attain economies of scale. As will be discussed later, some sterilisation procedures may be hazardous to human life if chemicals or radiation escape, so they have to be very carefully engineered to ensure worker safety; this can also be a significant capital and continuing financial burden on sterilisation facilities. Indeed, some jurisdictions have imposed environmental restrictions which may make it virtually impossible to operate in that jurisdiction. Many factors have to be considered in making a decision on the process to be used, to sterilise 'in-house' or by contract, and where to locate the facility.

Although not strictly a sterilisation process, aseptic processing is applied to some medical devices, e.g. solutions and some products which cannot withstand the conditions required by industrial sterilisation processes. Filtration of solutions through a $0.22 \mu m$ filter can effectively remove all microorganisms, but will not generally achieve the assurance levels required of terminally sterilised medical devices by EN 556.

## 5.2  THE STERILISATION PROCESS

### 5.2.1 GENERAL CONSIDERATIONS

There are three main methods used for large-scale industrial sterilisation: irradiation, ethylene oxide and moist heat. These can be further subdivided. Irradiation may be by gamma rays from cobalt-60 or caesium-137 radionuclides, or by electrons from an electron beam generator. Exposure to ethylene oxide in a sealed chamber may be to 100% ethylene oxide at subatmospheric pressures, or to gas mixtures including a chlorofluorocarbon (CFC), carbon dioxide or nitrogen, all at pressures well above atmospheric. Owing to restrictions on the use of CFCs in many parts of the world, the use of ethylene oxide mixtures with CFCs has generally been phased out.

Other methods are used by industry to a very minor extent and are usually employed because of some specific property of the device being sterilised. Dry heat, steam and formaldehyde, and glutaraldehyde all have some use and solutions may have to be handled using filtration or aseptic filling techniques because they cannot be subsequently sterilised. Experimental demonstration of other techniques, such as exposure to hydrogen peroxide, gas plasma, chlorine dioxide and ozone, has been reported (Health Industry Manufacturers Association, HIMA, 1988) but none seems to be making any headway against the three main procedures. X-rays have been demonstrated to sterilise surfaces but are not used routinely.

Sterilisation is usually carried out on devices in sealed packages (normally packed into cartons or corrugated card boxes, or both) as the last production stage of an otherwise 'ready-to-use' product. In an irradiator (gamma- or electron-beam) the packaged product is passed in front of the source of radiation, often two or possibly even four times, with different sides of the box facing the source in order to ensure that all the product is subject to a minimum dose. Ethylene oxide treatment is carried out in a sealed chamber for a time sufficient to allow the gas to penetrate all packaging material and the enclosed devices (where relevant), followed by the removal of residual gas. Steam treatment is carried out in an autoclave at a temperature in excess of $121\,°C$, the duration of treatment depending on the temperature, configuration and packaging of the device.

Safety is a prime concern of all managers of sterilisation facilities. Exposure to radiation and ethylene oxide gas can be lethal to humans. Even minor exposure to either can be very damaging. Access to gamma- or electron-beam irradiation chambers is carefully regulated. When not in use, the gamma source is stored in a water-filled pit, allowing safe access to the sterilisation bunker. In recent years more and more powerful generators have been designed to provide more energetic electrons for the purpose of giving higher penetration. However, a limit is imposed by the onset of induced radiation in some materials, and this must be covered in any qualification of an electron-beam process. Ethylene oxide is also an explosive gas, and an effort has been made to engineer non-explosive operating conditions using gas mixtures with only minor proportions of ethylene oxide (normally 6–12%). At the end of such a sterilisation cycle the residual gas is removed from the chamber and normally destroyed, either by conversion to relatively harmless dilute ethylene glycol, incineration or by a catalytic converter. Steam at temperatures greater than $121°C$ can also cause serious harm.

Each process has its advantages and disadvantages, usually dependent upon the composition of the device to be sterilised. Ethylene oxide exposure is usually carried out at temperatures of $20–50°C$ and is therefore ideal for plastics, especially those that have a relatively low melting temperature, e.g. polyvinyl chloride. Sterilisation chambers can treat a large quantity of product at any one time. However, the main disadvantages relate to the time required to penetrate and kill bacteria in complex or tortuous pathway devices, the difficulty of parametric release (release of product to the market based only on recorded physical parameters of the process), number of variables, need to use biological indicators (and the subsequent time required for testing them) and the potential residue of ethylene oxide left in the device after exposure. Some materials resist absorption of ethylene oxide and others can be desorbed fairly rapidly by heating and air washing. As a result of the deep vacuum or high pressure used in this type of sterilisation, great care must be taken to ensure that, whereas the packaging is porous to ethylene oxide, the seals maintaining sterility must be able to withstand the rate of pressure change imposed by the process.

Irradiation, particularly electron beam, can impose considerable constraints on the size of boxes that can be put through the system because penetration can fall off rapidly as a result of backscatter and energy absorption. Some modern facilities have addressed this issue and can process full-size pallets up to 2 m in height. Product density is a very important variable. Both gamma- and electron-beam radiation can cause considerable changes in plastics, e.g. discoloration, embrittlement, reduction in physical properties etc., but formulators have managed to reduce these effects in some plastics by means of additives, so that now many types of plastics can be irradiated. The process is also highly reproducible, so that physical indicators can be included in, or on, the boxes to demonstrate achievement of a minimum dose, 'read' immediately and hence the product released quickly for sale. Biological indicators are not required other than for qualifications or occasional spot checks. Recently published standards have allowed the introduction of dose-setting methods, opening up the possibility of lower doses being qualified. Previously a minimum dose of 25 kGy was fairly standard, but now devices with a very low bacterial load may be sterilised with a dose as low as half this value. This is important because it reduces the potential deleterious effect of the radiation on the materials in the device, and also reduces the maximum dose received by any device in the lot; by its nature the dose received will vary from unit to unit, depending on the distance from the source, backscatter etc., and a typical ratio of maximum:minimum dose found in any process is about 1.5. Absorption of radiation by materials may also cause a temperature rise of a few degrees, but this is not normally a problem.

Steam is a 'clean' sterilisation process with a predictable result. With minimum temperatures of 121°C required, it is severe on all plastics but is suitable for some textiles and is frequently used for equipment and devices made of metals or ceramics.

## 5.2.2 BIOLOGICAL INDICATORS

Some processes, e.g. irradiation, can be monitored by physical or chemical means. For others, e.g. ethylene oxide sterilisation, it is necessary to include biological monitors with the load during the process.

A biological monitor (indicator) is 'an inoculated carrier contained within its primary pack ready for use' (prEN 866 Part 1). The microorganisms selected for the indicator must be resistant to the sterilising process, i.e. at least as resistant as the most difficult to kill microorganism in the natural bioburden on the device. The indicator must be removed from the steriliser load as soon as possible after the end of the cycle and tested for viability, i.e. whether the organisms have all been killed or whether they are capable of metabolic activity or replication. This usually takes up to 7 days of incubation, and effectively means that the load cannot be released until after this time.

For ethylene oxide sterilisation the microorganism generally accepted for use in a biological indicator is *Bacillus subtilis* var. *niger* (NCTC 10073, ATCC 9372 or CIP 7718). For use with steam, *Bacillus stearothermophilus* (NCTC 1003, ATCC 7953, ATCC 12980 or CIP 5281) is suitable. If required for use with radiation, then *Bacillus pumilus* may be used, although it is not recommended practice to include biological indicators for radiation sterilisation.

## 5.2.3  PARAMETRIC RELEASE

Following completion of the manufacturing processes and any required testing, a designated responsible person must authorise release of the product for sale and use. For sterile products this includes an evaluation of all the sterilisation cycle parameters plus any biological testing required. Parametric release allows the responsible person to declare the product sterile based on physical and/or chemical process data alone, without any biological testing (of samples or biological indicators). For each sterilisation system, critical operating parameters (previously selected) must be met. Non-attainment of these parameters will preclude parametric release.

For irradiation, parametric release is possible using dosimeters which register the amount of radiation falling on them. Provided they are placed in locations which have been demonstrated to receive the minimum dose in the load, or in a reference location with a known relationship to the minimum dose, and the required minimum dose has been received, then the load can be assumed to have received the required dose to kill all microorganisms and can be released. Frequent dose audits are required to demonstrate the continued lethality of the minimum dose received.

Ethylene oxide cycles, on the other hand, have several variables (e.g. ethylene oxide concentration, temperature, exposure time, humidity in the load, possibly mixed load composition), all of which can effect the lethality of the cycle. It is therefore very difficult to set criteria for parametric release following an ethylene oxide cycle, and it is common practice to include biological indicators (monitors) in the cycle. Product release must then await confirmation that the microorganisms in the biological indicators have all been killed.

## 5.3  INDUSTRIAL PRODUCTION OF STERILE MEDICAL DEVICES

The actual sterilisation process is only the final step in a chain of planned systematic events designed by manufacturers to ensure product sterility. Equally, sterility is only one property required of many medical devices. Nevertheless, for those devices whose end-use requires a sterile product, the whole chain of events must be tightly controlled.

During design of the device, assuming that sterility is a required property, the manufacturer must decide what sterilisation process will be used. This may be dictated by facilities already owned or the decision may be open. The method of sterilisation will usually dictate (or be dictated by) the materials used in the device: can the materials withstand radiation, high temperatures etc.? The physical design of the device must be considered because penetration of gas through tortuous pathways may be very slow and is often a rate-determining factor. Some devices are designed to have a sterile fluid pathway but not necessarily a sterile exterior: this will affect the method of packaging.

Although the bacterial load (or bioburden) on a device (or batch of devices) will usually determine the extent of exposure to the sterilisation process (e.g. irradiation dose; gas concentration, temperature and time; steam temperature and exposure time), it is very important to reduce that exposure to an absolute minimum. This is not only to reduce potentially harmful effects to the device or its packaging during sterilisation, but also because the presence of numerous dead bacteria on a device can cause pyrogenicity and lead to other undesirable effects on a patient with a reduced immune system.

Hence the manufacturer must carry out operations in a 'clean room', i.e. a room with adequately filtered and controlled air circulation, and which is designed to reduce retention of bacteria and particulates, and for ease of cleaning, with operators appropriately dressed, with washed or covered hands. Standards (national and soon international) define clean rooms and clean air devices with different degrees of air cleanliness, and the manufacturer must decide the level of cleanliness appropriate to the device(s).

Raw materials and components should be controlled for bacterial contamination and manufacturing processes designed so that manual contact with the product and its component parts is minimised. The packaging that maintains the sterility of the device (the materials and sealing system) should be designed for ease of use and minimal handling.

All the above activities should form part of an integrated system. Often known as GMP (good manufacturing practice), this is now increasingly being aligned worldwide with the ISO 9001 standard (Quality system for assurance in design/development, production, installation and servicing), frequently supplemented by additional requirements specific to medical devices (e.g. EN 46001).

ISO 9001 (and 9002) were revised and reissued in 1994. EN 46001 (and EN 46002) were based on the 1987 versions of ISO 9001/2 and are being editorially revised to bring them into line with the 1994 versions. EN 724 is a guidance standard for non-active medical devices, providing suggestions on how manufacturers might meet the requirements in both ISO 9001/2 and EN 46001/2, but it also contains extensive guidance on the manufacture of sterile medical devices.

Recently ISO/TC 210 has been working to produce international standard versions of EN 46001/2, not simply as an endorsement of those standards, but as a technical revision incorporating input from non-CEN/CENELEC standards bodies. It is hoped that an ISO requirements standard for medical devices supplementing ISO 9001 can become, in effect, a 'global' GMP.

Having been manufactured under a quality system, in a clean room under controlled conditions with minimum handling, and sealed into a primary package, suitably labelled, the device is now ready for sterilisation. The quality system will have imposed microbiological control at appropriate points during manufacture and will provide a knowledge of the bacterial load to be sterilised.

Reproducibility and control of the entire manufacturing process is fundamental to the success of the sterilisation process in carrying out its function and delivering a guaranteed sterile product to the customer.

As the actual sterilisation process is one which cannot be assessed, either by inspection or by non-destructive testing, and because batch sterility testing proves nothing unless vast sample sizes are taken, the process needs qualification (i.e. demonstration that it is capable of fulfilling specified requirements, in this case providing a sterile product). The act of qualification is also referred to as 'process validation', but as already indicated in Chapter 2, the term validation is better reserved for products and the confirmation that they fulfil a specific intended use. Such methods of qualification for irradiation, ethylene oxide and moist steam processes have recently been set out clearly in standards, although it is useful to summarise the main points here.

Qualification covers two separate issues:

- the commissioning of the sterilisation apparatus and demonstration that it will achieve its intended purpose (i.e. killing bacteria)
- assurance that the specific sterilisation cycles selected will provide the sterility required, that the function of the product is not adversely affected, that packaging is robust enough to withstand the process, and finally that the management of the facility has reviewed the qualification and signed off all supporting documentation.

Standards also address the requirements for release of a product from quarantine following sterilisation. To this extent irradiation and steam have a definite advantage over ethylene oxide, which normally relies on incubation of biological indicators included with the devices in the process. Incubation normally takes 7 or more days, but release of the product can be earlier provided that the procedure has been fully qualified.

Most device manufacturing plants produce a variety of products, and frequently the steriliser must carry a heterogeneous load. The conditions of the cycle must therefore be set to cater for the most difficult to sterilise product in the load. This should be considered when setting the parameters in the cycle to be qualified for each product.

The method of sterilisation and whether to sterilise 'in house' or by contract with a specialist sterilisation company are decisions which, in the end, will largely be based on cost. Environmental and material issues may loom large, but they can be factored into the cost. How much will I have to pay for added engineering solutions to meet environmental requirements? If I select one method over another will I have to use more expensive materials? These days most contract sterilisers are registered to ISO 9001/2, and so their quality systems should be suitably adequate to cope with all requirements.

As the contract steriliser is treated as an extension of the manufacturing facility, the manufacturer must remain in control of the product until it is released for sale and not assume that the contractor will be responsible for everything. The sterilisation procedure may have an effect on the functionality of the device, and therefore during the product design, verification and/or validation phases (see ISO 9001:1994, Paragraphs 4.4.7 and 4.4.8) the manufacturer must demonstrate that the device, after sterilisation (and resterilisation one or more times, if allowed), meets its specification and performs as required.

During routine production, simulated use tests should be carried out at intervals on the sterilised product to ensure that no changes have inadvertently occurred. Also, any material or process change in production should be investigated to see whether it may affect the functionality of the device after sterilisation. Resterilisation should also be qualified. Irradiation of a device is a cumulative experience and, although one exposure may be acceptable, double that exposure may cause considerable material change. Ethylene oxide is usually much more gentle to the device but repeated cycling through vacuum or high-pressure stages may put an intolerable strain on sterile package seals, or indeed cause material damage to the device. If the materials of the device are susceptible to retention of ethylene oxide residue, then resterilisation may cause intolerably high residues to be retained.

## 5.4 HOSPITAL STERILISATION

Most sterilisation carried out by hospital departments employs moist heat, although some hospitals have small ethylene oxide sterilisers. Much of the sterilisation relates to reusable surgical instruments and wrapped loads. However, some is carried out on temperature-sensitive materials and on devices which have been heavily contaminated, and some is carried out on a 'one-off' basis and on single-use devices in an effort to reuse them.

Compared to industrial sterilisation, where the devices have a low bioburden and are made from virgin materials that are well characterised and whose response to the sterilisation process has been qualified, hospital steriliser managers face a much more difficult task. Contaminated products must be put through a qualified cleaning system prior to sterilisation. Sophisticated and qualified packaging equipment will not normally be available. Especially when trying to reuse single-use devices, the material characteristics will not be known. When using ethylene oxide in 'one-off' situations, there is no possibility of process qualification. By the nature of the work, sterilisation loads will be of a very heterogeneous nature. All this points to the difficulties experienced in running a hospital steriliser or sterilisation department, and the considerable risks of there being non-sterile devices or ones with reduced functionality.

Although reusable surgical instruments (such as forceps or scissors) are not normally sold with advice on how many times they can be resterilised, the conditions during moist heat sterilisation are quite severe and even these devices will deteriorate with time, and should be checked for functionality at appropriate intervals.

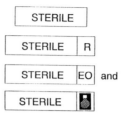

**Figure 5.2**   CEN symbols for (a) 'Sterile'; (b) 'Sterile' by radiation method; (c) 'Sterile' by ethylene oxide; (d) 'Sterile' by steam or dry heat

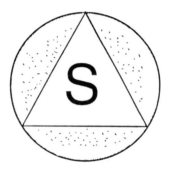

**Figure 5.3**   ISO pictogram symbol for 'sterile'

## 5.5   LABELLING

Labelling is frequently a regulatory issue and contains information that the manufacturer wishes to impart to the user. With increasing worldwide regulation of medical devices (frequently requiring local language to provide information or instructions for use) a symbol for 'sterile' is a useful adjunct for manufacturers. In Europe, CEN has proposed a symbol in prEN 980, with additional symbols covering the sterilisation method (Figure 5.2).

However, although these may be acceptable in Europe, where English is a widely used commercial language and 'sterile' in many other languages is only a minor variation on the English word, there may well be difficulty in gaining acceptability for such symbols in countries which do not use Roman letters or understand English. Hence a more pictogram-type symbol has been proposed by an ISO committee (Figure 5.3), but a the final choice has not yet been made.

## 5.6   RESIDUALS

### 5.6.1   GENERAL CONSIDERATIONS

During the manufacture of medical devices the materials used may come into contact with liquids or gases that may be absorbed into, or on to, the finished device. In particular, when using ethylene oxide for sterilisation, the gas may be absorbed into the material and may react to form ethylene chlorohydrin or ethylene glycol. As a rule, it is most unlikely that sufficient ethylene glycol will be formed to provide any significant risk, but at least on an acute basis ethylene chlorohydrin may be more toxic than ethylene oxide.

According to the International Agency for Research on Cancer (IARC, 1996), whereas 'there is limited evidence in humans for the carcinogenicity of ethylene oxide, there is sufficient evidence in experimental animals for its carcinogenicity' and their overall evaluation is that 'ethylene oxide is a Group 1 carcinogen to humans'. Thus although ethylene oxide is a very effective sterilant for medical devices, its toxicity on exposure to patients and health service personnel must be borne in mind. Historically there have been attempts to limit the amount of ethylene oxide in devices, either by Pharmacopoeia (e.g. French, Italian, European) or by draft regulations (e.g. USA, Germany). These have not always been enforced, and most other countries have not felt any real need to regulate ethylene oxide residues.

However, as already indicated in Chapter 2, the EU medical devices Directive (93/42/EEC) has an essential requirement in Annex 1 which says 'devices must be designed and manufactured in such a way as to reduce to a minimum the risks posed by substances leaking from the device'. 'Leaking' in this context is taken to include the transfer of substances such as ethylene oxide from the device to the patient. The term 'to a minimum' should also be noted: it does not mean eliminate, thereby allowing for the benefit to the patient of, for example, the availability of a sterile device at a reasonable cost even if it has some residual ethylene oxide, provided that the risk has been minimised as far as possible.

In order to provide indications of acceptable limits for ethylene oxide (and ethylene chlorohydrin) in medical devices, ISO/TC 194 WG 11 (Ethylene oxide sterilisation residues) has formulated a standard which is expected to be published shortly as ISO 10993 (EN 30993), Part 7. Following the guidance of ISO 10993-1, devices were divided into limited exposure (single or multiple use or contact of less than 24 hours), prolonged exposure (single, multiple or long-term use, or contact of 24 hours to 30 days) and permanent contact (single, multiple or long-term use, or contact exceeding 30 days). Limits were then set, based on all the existing known risk-based studies, for each category. The limits were set on a daily dose to the patient, with compliance based on extracting the residue using a simulated use method and measuring the quantity of residue extracted. Alternatively, and especially if no validated simulated use method is available, if the residue is under the limit when tested by an exhaustive extraction method, this will also be acceptable. The limits for the various category of devices are as follows:

- For limited exposure, the average daily dose to patient shall not exceed 20 mg/day ethylene oxide or 12 mg/day ethylene chlorohydrin.
- For prolonged exposure, the average daily dose to patient shall not exceed 2 mg/day ethylene oxide (with a maximum of 20 mg in the first 24 hours and

60 mg in the first 30 days) and 2 mg/day ethylene chlorohydrin (with a maximum of 12 mg in the first 24 hours and 60 mg in the first 30 days).
- For permanent contact, the average daily dose to patient shall not exceed 0.1 mg/day ethylene oxide (with a maximum of 20 mg in the first 24 hours, 60 mg in the first 30 days and 2.5 g in a lifetime) and 2 mg/day for ethylene chlorohydrin (with a maximum of 12 mg in the first 24 hours, 60 mg in 30 days and 50 g in a lifetime).

In arriving at these limits the expert WG allowed some exceptions:

- For multidevice systems, the limits shall apply to each device.
- For intraocular lenses, ethylene oxide shall not exceed 0.5 mg/lens/day, nor 1.25 mg/lens.
- For blood oxygenators and blood separators, the average daily dose of ethylene oxide to patient shall not exceed 60 mg.
- For extracorporeal blood purification set-ups the ethylene oxide and ethylene chlorohydrin limits for the prolonged and limited categories apply, but the lifetime limit for ethylene oxide may be exceeded.

Although these limits passed the voting requirements in both CEN and ISO, certain reservations were expressed, especially for devices which may be used frequently, devices used on neonates and small children, devices used simultaneously, and kits of several devices used in one procedure and for populations at high risk. For these and other reasons, the standard has immediately been entered for revision. In order to assist that revision, the same ISO WG is preparing another standard (to become ISO 14538) which will provide a methodology for setting residue limits for any molecular species in a medical device using a health-based risk assessment approach. When the methodology is sufficiently accepted, it will then be applied to ethylene oxide, ethylene chlorohydrin (and ethylene glycol) to decide whether the limits set in ISO 10993-7 do indeed require such revision. To date, no standard has been proposed for residues of glutaraldehyde or formaldehyde, but there is probably only a small minority of devices that are sterilised using these chemicals.

One further point should be borne in mind by those using radiation to sterilise medical devices. Radiation can cause degradation in materials (especially plastics) and can cause chemical reactions to produce species differing from the original materials. Irradiated devices should be investigated during design validation to ensure that the radiation has not caused or led to the appearance of residues of toxic or carcinogenic chemicals.

Whether a device absorbs and/or retains ethylene oxide depends to a very large extent on the materials used: soft plastics normally absorb more than hard; metals or ceramics will not normally absorb ethylene oxide; a source of free chlorine ions may well catalyse the conversion of ethylene oxide to ethylene chlorohydrin. Some materials may absorb ethylene oxide easily, but also retain it very strongly, so that very little may be released to the patient. Sterilisation cycles using high ethylene oxide concentrations, long exposure times or elevated temperatures will probably cause higher residue levels. However, each device type and each sterilisation cycle has to be treated as a separate case, and it is almost impossible to predict the behaviour of the 'system' prior to testing. Residual ethylene oxide can generally be reduced or practically eliminated by forced aeration. The rate of removal is a complex function of many variables, e.g. load density, temperature, air flow, time and the surface:volume ratio of the device.

### 5.6.2  MEASUREMENT OF RESIDUAL ETHYLENE OXIDE IN DEVICES

In deciding whether a certain amount of ethylene oxide in, or on, a device is 'safe', it is necessary to determine how much of any ethylene oxide present will contact or enter the patient. A simple measure of the 'total' ethylene oxide content is not necessary, but may be the easiest determination analytically and, provided it is below the safe limit, may be all that is required. However, for most devices only a fraction of the ethylene oxide present will actually contact the patient. This may be due to one of several reasons, e.g. the device may only be used in contact with the patient for a very short time; the material may strongly retain ethylene oxide; and the method of contact may not be particularly sensitive.

Determination of the amount of ethylene oxide in a device that will transfer to the patient therefore becomes a two-step problem:

- development of a validated, 'simulated-use' extraction method that accurately mimics the route of transfer of ethylene oxide from the device to the patient
- measurement of the actual amount of ethylene oxide extracted.

The ISO standard 10993-7 provides guidance on both simulated-use and 'total' extraction, together with suggested methods to measure the quantity of ethylene oxide extracted. More sensitive methods are currently being developed and will be included in future revisions of the standard.

## 5.7  STANDARDS

Although there have been national standards covering various aspects of sterilisation and sterilisers and disinfectors, it is only recently that concerted efforts have been made to harmonise texts internationally to provide consensus standards. CEN established its TC 204 (Sterilisation of medical devices) in 1989 and ISO followed by setting up its TC 198 shortly thereafter. The impetus behind the formation of CEN/TC 204 was the need to provide standards for sterilisation procedures to support the European Directives then being written for active implantable medical devices (90/385/EEC) and medical devices in general (93/42/EEC). ISO/TC 198 was formed largely to provide a wider international forum and, although liaison between the two committees (and CEN/TC 102 relating to sterilisers and related accessories) has been good and there has been

**Table 5.1** Process standards

| | |
|---|---|
| ISO 11134:1994 | Requirements for validation and routine control – industrial moist heat sterilisation |
| ISO 11135:1994 | Validation and routine control of ethylene oxide sterilisation |
| ISO 11137:1995 | Requirements for validation and routine control – radiation sterilisation |
| ISO/DIS 13683 | Requirements for validation and routine control – moist heat sterilisation in healthcare facilities |
| ISO/DIS 14160* | Validation and routine control of sterilisation of single-use medical devices incorporating materials of animal origin by liquid chemical sterilants |
| ISO/CD 13408 | Aseptic processing of healthcare products |
| ISO/CD 13409 | Substantiation of 25 kGy for radiation sterilisation of small or infrequent production batches |
| ISO/WD 14724 | Dose setting using the radiation resistance of microbial isolates |
| ISO/NP* | General criteria for sterilisation processes |
| EN 550:1994 | Validation and routine control of ethylene oxide sterilisation |
| EN 552:1994 | Validation and routine control of sterilisation by irradiation |
| EN 554:1994 | Validation and routine control of sterilisation by moist heat |

*Also on the CEN work programme
Note: CEN/TC 204 is proposing standards on:
• aseptic processing of medical devices
• information to be provided by the supplier for the reprocessing of resterilisable devices – requirements.

much in common, there are also some differences of opinion and approaches. For instance, CEN has felt obliged to define a practical means of deciding whether a device may be labelled 'sterile' or not, whereas ISO leaves the process end-point up to regulators. A more major point of divergence lies in the respective scopes of the standards: ISO/TC 198 covers sterilisation of healthcare products, which is wider than CEN/TC 204's scope of sterilisation of medical devices.

EN 556 (Requirements for medical devices to be labelled 'sterile') generated considerable discussion during drafting and continues to be a divergent issue. It requires a maximum chance of 1 in $10^6$ of a device being non-sterile. prEN 980 is proposing to tie the use of the CEN symbol for 'sterile' (Figure 5.2) to the requirement in EN 556.

It is generally felt, however, that the requirement in EN 556 is unnecessarily strict for some devices, e.g. non-invasive devices. CEN/TC 204 took the position that 'sterile' can only have one meaning: a device is either sterile or it is not, and it cannot be 'semisterile'. As the absolute property of sterility cannot be readily proven, the criteria in EN 556 is based on probability. Considerable thought and discussion has taken place on alternative terms to indicate, for instance, a maximum chance of non-sterility of 1 in $10^3$, with no success to date. The fact that prEN 980 proposes to use the word 'sterile' in a box as a symbol also causes problems outside Europe. ISO guidelines indicate that words cannot be symbols (no language is universal), and a pictogram may be more readily understood. This opens the possibility of there being different standard symbols for 'sterile' in

Table 5.2   Accessory standards

| | |
|---|---|
| ISO 11138-1:1994 | Biological indicators – 1: general requirements |
| ISO 11138-2:1994 | Biological indicators – 2: ethylene oxide sterilisation |
| ISO 11138-3:1994 | Biological indicators – 3: moist heat sterilisation |
| ISO 11140-1:1995 | Chemical indicators – 1: general requirements |
| ISO/WD 11140-2 | Chemical indicators – 2: test methods |
| ISO/CD 11140-3 | Chemical indicators – 3: requirements for Bowie–Dick indicators |
| ISO/DIS 11607 | Packaging for terminally sterilised medical devices |
| ISO 11737-1 | Microbiological methods – 1: estimation of the population of microorganisms on products |
| ISO/DIS 11737-2 | Microbiological methods – 2: tests for sterility performed in the validation of a sterilisation process |
| ISO/NP 14161 | Guidance on the use of biological indicators in validation and routine control |
| prEN 1174-1 | Estimation of the population of microorganisms on product – 1: requirements |
| prEN 1174-2 | Estimation of the population of microorganisms on product – 2: guidance |
| prEN 1174-3 | Estimation of the population of microorganisms on product – 3: guidance to the methods of validation of microbiological techniques |
| proposed EN1174-4 | Estimation of the population of microorganisms on product – 4: statistical model |
| prEN 866-1* | Biological systems for testing sterilisers – 1: general requirements |
| prEN 866-2* | Biological systems for testing sterilisers – 2: ethylene oxide |
| prEN 866-3* | Biological systems for testing sterilisers – 3: moist heat requirements |
| prEN 867-1 | Non-biological systems for use in sterilisers – 1: general requirements |
| prEN 867-2 | Non-biological systems for use in sterilisers – 2: process indicators (class A) |
| prEN 867-3 | Non-biological systems for use in sterilisers – 3: Class B indicators for the Bowie–Dick test |
| proposed EN 867-4 | Non-biological systems for use in sterilisers – 4: systems equivalent to the Bowie–Dick test |
| proposed EN 867-5 | Non-biological systems for use in sterilisers – 5: multivariable systems for Class B sterilisers |
| prEN 868-1** | Packing materials – 1: general requirements and tests |

\* Note: EN 866 is proposed to include at least five more parts covering other biological indicator systems
\*\* Note: EN 868 is proposed to include at least 10 more parts covering various packaging materials
Note: CEN/TC 102 is proposing standards on:
• use of sterilising accessories
• guidance on packaging materials for sterilisation of wrapped goods.

Europe and the rest of the world. However, the proposal currently being discussed for an ISO 'sterile' symbol is not readily understood and would probably require a major training effort to teach healthcare professionals its meaning.

**Table 5.3** Sterilisers/washer disinfectors

| | |
|---|---|
| prEN 285 | Steam sterilisers – large |
| proposed EN | Steam sterilisers – small: requirements and testing |
| prEN 1422 | Ethylene oxide sterilisers – specification |
| proposed EN | Mode of use and maintenance of sterilisers |
| proposed EN | Washer disinfectors – general requirements, definitions and tests |
| proposed EN | Washer disinfectors – for surgical instruments and trays, anaesthetic equipment, hollowware and glassware |
| proposed EN | Washer disinfectors – for human waste containers |

**Table 5.4** General standards

| | |
|---|---|
| EN 556:1994 | Requirements for medical devices to be labelled 'sterile' |
| EN ISO 10993-7 | Biological evaluation of medical devices – 7: ethylene oxide sterilisation residuals |
| prEN 980 | Graphic symbols for use in the labelling of medical devices |
| ISO/CD 14538 | Method for the establishment of allowable limits for residues in medical devices using health-based risk assessment |

**Table 5.5** Other standards

| | |
|---|---|
| EN ISO 9001:1994 | Quality systems – model for quality assurance in design, development, production, installation and servicing |
| EN ISO 9002:1994 | Quality systems – model for quality assurance in production, installation and servicing |
| EN 46001:1993 | Quality systems – medical devices: particular requirements for the application of EN ISO 9001 |
| EN 46002:1993 | Quality systems – medical devices: particular requirements for the application of EN ISO 9002 |
| EN 724:1994 | Guidance on the application of EN ISO 9001 and EN 46001 and of EN ISO 9002 and EN 46002 for non-active medical devices |
| EN ISO 8402:1994 | Quality management and quality assurance – vocabulary |
| ISO/DIS 13485 | Quality systems – medical devices: particular requirements for the application of EN ISO 9001 |
| ISO/DIS 13488 | Quality systems – medical devices: particular requirements for the application of EN ISO 9002 |

All the relevant CEN and ISO standards, both published and in various stages of production, are summarised in Tables 5.1–5.5.

## 5.8   THE FUTURE

What does the future hold? It would appear that there is no 'new' method of sterilisation 'just around the corner' to challenge irradiation, ethylene oxide and steam. Dry heat, low-temperature steam and formaldehyde, and glutaraldehyde will hold some attractions for particular materials/devices, and steam will continue to be the method of choice for hospitals, and doctors' and dental surgeries.

Environmental issues will play an increasing part in deciding future investment in sterilisation facilities. Attempts will continue to be made by vested interests to demonstrate that one or other method is cheapest. Safety of plant personnel and patients is of prime concern, and strict control of possible exposure to either radiation or ethylene oxide must be exercised. Venting of ethylene oxide to the atmosphere, with consequent possible exposure of local populations, must also be avoided, although local planning laws and regulations in most countries will ensure that this risk is virtually non-existent.

Standards, either published or near publication, by both CEN and ISO will have a dramatic effect in improving confidence in sterile devices in those countries subject to strong regulation, by virtue of opening the qualification and routine control of sterilisation processes to third-party audit. For those countries already subject to such control, the published methods should remove a number of contentious issues.

Probably the single most important issue that will continue to exercise industrial managers will be whether to sterilise 'in house' or contract out. In recent years the trend has been to contract out, especially when product volumes are low, and this is likely to continue. The capital cost of sterilisation facilities will favour dedicated sterilisation companies, which can achieve savings by increasing throughput and utilisation and which can also shoulder the burden of complying with all environmental requirements.

The debate on what should be required of a product in order to label it 'sterile' will continue, with advocates of the position taken by EN 556 and those of a more flexible approach voicing their opinions.

## 5.9  REFERENCES

HIMA (1988) Sterilisation in the1990s. HIMA Conf. Proc., Washington DC, USA.
IARC (1996) Ethylene oxide. IARC monograph report, 60:73–159.
Morrisey RF and Briggs G (eds.) (1993) Sterilisation technology: a practical guide for manufacturers and users of health-care products. Phillips–van Nostrand Reinhold, Amsterdam, The Netherlands.

# 6

# Cytotoxicity

# Part I: Toxicological Risk Evaluation Using Cell Culture

MARIE-FRANÇOISE HARMAND
Laboratoire d'Evaluation des Matériels Implantables, Martillac, France

## 6.1  INTRODUCTION

As indicated in Chapter 2, biocompatibility has been defined as 'the ability of a material to perform with an appropriate host response in a specific application' (Williams, 1991). It is through the design process of a medical device that evaluation of biocompatibility is made in order to provide assurance that the final device will be safe for human use and perform as intended.

During the past 30 years this evaluation has been carried out *in vivo* using animals (rats, rabbits, dogs, sheep etc.) according to the recommendations of a variety of standard organisations. However, such tests are expensive, time-consuming and likely to be limited for ethical reasons. The ISO standard 10993-2 (Biological evaluation of medical devices, Part 2: Animal welfare requirements) recommends that 'animal experiments shall not be performed before appropriate tests, if available, have been carried out'.

For these reasons *in vitro* tests based on cell culture were established in order to evaluate cytotoxicity:

- in research and development for the screening of innovative materials
- for the initial testing of medical devices
- for the quality control of products (raw materials or final devices).

Cytotoxicity can be defined as the '*in vitro* evaluation of toxicological risks using cell culture'. Thus the concept of cytotoxicity may be developed on a large scale, from cell viability and death to a more sophisticated approach dealing with cell functionality and genotoxicity (see Chapter 8 for a detailed discussion of this and related biological responses), since toxic substances arising from biomaterials

*Biocompatibility Assessment of Medical Devices and Materials.*
Edited by Julian Braybrook. © 1997 John Wiley & Sons Ltd.

interact at the cellular level with cell membranes, cell organelles (mitochondria and liposomes), protein synthesis, DNA synthesis and cell division, and DNA sequences. These substances arise from:

• additives, process contaminants and residues
• leachable substances
• biodegradation products.

Moreover, material surface chemistry (the detection techniques for which have already been discussed in Chapter 4) can also alter cell membrane functionality.

Until recently, cytotoxicity studies have been limited to qualitative or semiquantitative tests using either established, transformed or neoplastic cell lines. The progress achieved in the last few years, associated with the culture of mammalian cells, has allowed the development of quantitative assays for cytotoxicity assessment which are highly reproducible and sensitive.

## 6.2   ISO 10993 (EN 30993), PART 5: TESTS FOR CYTOTOXICITY – *IN VITRO* METHODS

### 6.2.1   INTRODUCTION

In the framework of ISO/TC 194, it is WG5 which has been working to prepare a cytotoxicity standard. Its initial objective was to harmonise existing national and international standards (ASTM, 1983, 1984; AS, 1984; ISO, 1984; NFS, 1988a; BS, 1988, 1989; PAB, 1989; FDA, 1989; USP, 1990; DIN, 1990). However, WG5 also had the objective of taking into account the recent progress achieved in cell culturing and to focus on the quantitative evaluation of cell cytotoxicity.

### 6.2.2   TEST PROCEDURES

Cytotoxicity is evaluated through the following types of tests:

• contact with specific liquid extracts prepared from the material
• direct contact with the final device or samples of the final device precursors
• indirect contact (diffusion) with either liquid extracts or solid materials.

The choice as to which type of test should be performed depends on the material and its intended use.

#### 6.2.2.1   Test on Extract

The liquid extract of a test material is obtained by immersing the material in an extractant (preferably serum-free mammalian cell culture medium or serum-supplemented cell culture medium) in an incubator at 37°C for not less than 24 hours, using a material surface area (or weight):extractant volume of 3–6 cm$^2$/ml

(0.1–0.2 g/ml). The original liquid extract and several of its dilutions (50%, 10%, 1%) are assessed for cytotoxicity in triplicate after varying time intervals (24 h, 48 h, 72 h) in contact with near-confluent monolayers of the selected cell line.

### 6.2.2.2  Test by Direct Contact

A sample of the test material is placed in the centre of a near-confluent monolayer of the selected cell line so that it covers one-tenth of the cell layer. Cytotoxicity is again evaluated in triplicate after varying time intervals (24 h, 48 h, 72 h).

### 6.2.2.3  Test by Indirect Contact (Diffusion)

*Agar overlay*

A sample of the test material is placed on a solidified agar/culture medium mixture covering a near-confluent monolayer of the selected cell line. Cytotoxicity is evaluated in triplicate after a 24-hour incubation period.

*Filter diffusion*

The selected cell line is grown to near confluence on surfactant-free filters (0.45 $\mu$m pore size). The filters are then transferred, cell side down, on to a layer of solidified agar/culture medium mixture. Test materials are placed on the acellular (top) side of the filter. Cytotoxicity is evaluated in triplicate after a 24-hour incubation period.

### 6.2.3  *DETERMINATION OF CYTOTOXICITY*

### 6.2.3.1  Test on Extract or by Direct Contact

These tests allow both qualitative and quantitative evaluation of cytotoxicity. They can be a measure of cell death, inhibition of cell proliferation, amount of protein, release of enzymes or other measurable parameter.

### 6.2.3.2  Test by Indirect Contact (Diffusion)

These tests only allow a semiquantitative evaluation of cytotoxicity based on morphological observation, using the uptake of a vital stain (e.g. neutral red), with respect to the diameter of the decolorised area (i.e. zone index) and percentage of dead cells within this area (i.e. lysis index). Furthermore, in the agar overlay test the overlay may limit diffusion of toxic substances from the test material to the cell layer, thereby giving rise to false negative results. It should be carefully noted, therefore, that cytotoxicity is heavily dependent on the composition and thickness of the agar barrier in this test.

*6.2.4   CELL LINES*

Established cell lines from recognised repositories are preferred, e.g. L929, Balb/C 3T3, MRC5, HeLa etc. Primary cell cultures and cell lines obtained from mammalian tissues can be used if specific sensitivity is required. In all cases the cell lines must be free from mycoplasma.


*6.2.5   CONTROL MATERIALS*

Negative (i.e. non-cytotoxic) and positive (i.e. a reproducible cytotoxic response) control materials must be run in parallel with the test material(s) in each test. Such liquid materials include silver solutions as positive controls; solid control materials include (but are by no means limited to) low-density polyethylene (e.g. US origin), and doped polyvinyl chloride (e.g. UK origin) or doped polyurethane (e.g. Japanese origin) respectively. These matrices are not, however, certified reference materials and should not be mistaken for such.


## 6.3   CRITICAL ANALYSIS OF ISO 10993-5

This standard represents synthesis and harmonisation of various pre-existing standards on the one hand, and on the other takes into account new concepts in the evaluation of cytotoxicity, mainly quantitative assessment of cytotoxicity and the use of primary cell culture (and cell lines) arising from mammalian tissues.

Quantitative assessment produces objective data highly amenable to statistical treatment and precise kinetics analysis, if necessary. In the framework of well-standardised test procedures, established cell lines have the advantages of high reproducibility of test results and low cost, and may be used routinely in the screening stage of cytotoxicity testing when cell functions shared by all cell types are to be considered (i.e. cell viability, cell membrane integrity, mitosis etc.) because these cell lines are poorly differentiated and mainly involved in replication.

In the field of biocompatibility assessment it is most desirable that *in vitro* cytotoxicity testing should have some clinical relevance. Thus the emerging use of mammalian cells will potentially allow such an evaluation of functional cytocompatibility of materials (NFS, 1988b–f and 1989a–e). The modification of specific metabolic functions can then be evaluated using mammalian cell systems arising from the tissue belonging to the future site of implantation of the material/device (Harmand *et al.*, 1986). As indicated in the standard, measurable parameters which are related to cell phenotype expression may be quantified, for example using human osteoblasts, cytotoxicity will be assessed through cell viability together with the study of cell growth and cellular alkaline phosphatase activity (Naji and Harmand, 1991). This interesting opening to cell lines arising from mammalian tissues implies that these cell lines should preferably be used provided that their reproducibility and accuracy of response can be demonstrated.

Thus their use is to be recommended as a second-intention test in an attempt to obtain an evaluation of biocompatibility (cytocompatibility), and propose an alternative method to animal experimentation. This approach also needs to be assessed in the framework of interlaboratory programmes taking into consideration the correlation with preclinical and clinical test results.

*In vitro* toxicity testing is a technically complicated activity and many sources of error or artefact exist which can lead to erroneous conclusions. It is recommended that personnel involved in cytotoxicity testing of medical devices be adequately trained in cell culture procedures and basic toxicology. Preferably this should be under constant review, and even form part of third-party accreditation, e.g. ISO 9000 (EN 45000) series etc.

The biological component of cytotoxicity testing systems must be fully characterised, e.g. tissue source, passage number, absence of mycoplasma etc. In the case of primary cell cultures or cell lines arising from living tissues it is necessary to focus on the purity of the cell preparation and representative cellular characteristics. The pH and the osmolarity of the liquid extract are important characteristics that need to be measured, as they too can influence the behaviour of cells. Hence during direct contact testing, the pH should lie in the range 6.5–8.0 and osmolarity should be *ca.* 350 mmol/l. If antimicrobial or antifungal agents are used, a concentration–response curve for these agents should also be reported. Furthermore, alterations in the culture medium may occur owing to reactions between the serum and cell culture medium and the liquid extract or test material, e.g. serum protein denaturation or adsorption, alteration of nutrients etc. Interaction between serum proteins and toxic elements may artificially reduce or increase the level of cytotoxicity by respectively inhibiting or facilitating cellular uptake. Thus it should be noted that the amount of serum needs to be considered carefully, and two different concentrations of serum are commonly used to palliate this possible effect.

When working with an extract, quantitation of the actual dosage to the culture of each constituent of the original test material should be very useful, but is difficult.

A critical point in the evaluation of *in vitro* cytotoxicity is the difficulty of interpreting data generated in its study with respect to the clinical use of the medical device, taking into account the risks and benefits. This issue is considered in more detail in Chapter 10.

## 6.4 CONCLUSIONS

The acquisition of reproducible cytotoxicity data is certainly feasible through the use of ISO 10993-5 (EN 30993-5), provided that the potential technical problems are adequately taken into account and that the performance of the test system is carefully monitored. This implies that cytotoxicity testing should be performed by specialised personnel, in a rigorous standardised manner working in compliance with EN 45001.

Future work will be developed in order to produce precise standardisation of various cytotoxicity testing procedures to deal with medical devices from diverse clinical interests.

As already indicated in Chapter 2, there are at present no 'biological' certified reference materials, CRMs. The aforementioned control and other like materials have not undergone the rigorous collaborative testing and certification required and, even though they are commonly mistaken as being CRMs, they are not. Indeed, a much wider selection of matrices with properties more relevant to the specific test material(s) is required, particularly for cytotoxicity testing purposes. A number are currently in development and it is proposed by key WG5 members active in this area to feed these into as international a collaborative study as possible to produce CRMs, while also investigating the further standardisation of each of the current cytotoxicity tests described above with a view to prioritising them and, in the future, producing critical end-points for the tests where possible.

# Part II: Apoptosis

ROSY ELOY AND N. WEILL
Biomatech, Chasse-sur-Rhône, France

## 6.5   INTRODUCTION

Apoptosis, or programmed cell death, is a sequence of intracellular events (under physiological conditions) that lead to cell death (Krammer et al., 1994; Majno and Joris, 1995). It has been shown that apoptosis:

- is a necessary mechanism in certain physiological conditions, e.g. embryogenesis, homeostasis of the immune system, erythropoiesis etc.
- serves as a major mechanism for the precise regulation of cell numbers
- serves as a defence mechanism to remove self-active lymphocytes and tumour cells.

Some xenobiotics can induce apoptosis at lower doses and oncosis (some researchers still refer to this form of cell death as necrosis) at higher doses; the two processes have distinct differences in their characteristics (see the following section).

Once triggered, apoptosis starts with a reversible precommitment phase during which a high level of secondary messengers (e.g. calcium, $IP_3$ and/or cAMP) is observable in the cell. An irreversible commitment phase then follows (even if the trigger source is removed), unless forcibly suppressed, e.g. by inhibition of the synthesis of the macromolecules required. As a result, several characteristic morphological and biochemical changes are observable.

## 6.6 KEY FEATURES OF THE PROCESS

The key features of apoptosis are:

* morphological changes
  The cell shrinks and becomes a denser, more rounded mass (as implied by the original name of shrinkage necrosis). The chromatin becomes pyknotic and packed into smooth masses marginalised to the nuclear membrane, thereby creating curved profiles (which have inspired such descriptive terms as half-moon, horseshoe, sickle, lancet and ship-like/navicular) and breaking up the nucleus (karyolysis), so causing the cell to emit processes (the budding phenomenon) which often contain pyknotic nuclear fragments (which tend to break off as apoptotic bodies themselves and remain free or are phagocytosed by macrophages or neighbouring cells). There is little or no resulting swelling (inflammatory response) of mitochondria or other organelles.
* biochemical changes
  The activation of an endonuclease causes the DNA to break down into fragments of 180–200 base pairs, or multiples of *ca.* 185 base pairs, and subsequently into very small oligonucleosomal fragments. The destruction of the DNA is actually the first event during apoptosis, lysis of the plasma membrane being the last.
* the process is genetically controlled and can be initiated by an internal clock or extracellular agents, e.g. hormones, cytokines, killer cells, and a variety of chemical, physical and viral agents.
* the process can run its course very quickly, even in minutes, from the onset of budding to complete break-up, and so remains unobtrusive in tissue sections. In routine sections the best cytological marker of apoptosis is karyolysis, especially in an isolated cell. Fortunately, a recent histochemical advance, which uses the fact that DNA breaking points (nicks) expose chemically specific molecular endings, enables the simple identification of apoptosis.

However, cell suicide does not always take the form of apoptosis: cell murder by cytotoxic lymphocytes leads to apoptosis. Furthermore, there appear to be several varieties of apoptosis and different cell types may follow different rules.

The above features should be differentiated from those related to oncosis (formerly necrosis), or catastrophic/accidental cell death, which occurs when cells are exposed to extreme variation from physiological conditions and results in damage to the plasma membrane. Its particular characteristics are:

* morphological changes
  There is an increase in the plasma membrane permeability, and cellular swelling, organelle swelling and vacuolisation, and simultaneous protein denaturation and hydrolysis are observable. Intracellular contents are released into the extracellular fluid and this, *in vivo*, is often associated with extensive tissue damage (resulting in a fibrous scar) and an intense inflammatory

response. The increased membrane permeability allows diagnosis of activation of this process by tests based on dye exclusion or electron microscopy with colloidal markers.

- biochemical changes
  The DNA breaks down, post-lytically, in a non-specific/random fashion.
- the process typically arises as a result of hypothermia, hypoxia, ischaemia, and possibly toxic agents that interfere with ATP (adenosine triphosphate) generation or cause failure of the membrane's ionic pumps
- the process evolves within 24 hours to typical necrosis
- it is usually accompanied by karyolysis.

## 6.7  RELATIONSHIP TO CYTOTOXICITY

It has been hypothesised that cell transformation could be due to a sudden resistance to apoptosis. However, it has recently been demonstrated that well known anticancer drugs are able to induce apoptosis. Several genes have been reported to be associated with programmed cell death; pathological processes appear as a consequence of apoptosis suppression, some of the responsible genes having been identified, e.g. oncogene *bcl*-2 in human follicular B-cell lymphoma.

The consequence of apoptosis for studying cell–material interactions is therefore that the very early signs of induction to apoptosis should be looked for in order to better define cytotoxicity. Attention should also be paid to oncosis (formerly necrosis).

## 6.8  RELATIONSHIP TO MUTAGENICITY/CARCINOGENICITY

Even though mutagenicity/carcinogenicity is discussed later in this book (Chapter 8), it is more relevant to discuss any relationship with apoptosis here.

Apoptosis and tumour development may be related, as both are regulated by transcription factors. When DNA is damaged, the gene product p53 is expressed. Its function can be summarised as being a checkpoint for the cell cycle, leading either to cell cycle arrest (with DNA repair) or cell death (through apoptosis). p53 appears to be required predominantly for mediating the apoptotic response to chromosomal damage, and is therefore placed in an activation pathway upstream of the basic cell death programme. Without its expression, the cell may continue to replicate (including its damaged DNA) and, through a multistage development, neoplasia may develop. In contrast to oncogene mutations, which are dominant, mutations to the p53 gene are recessive. Considering that about 70% of tumours have some sort of defect in p53, it is evident that this molecule has an important decisive function in cell cycle regulation. The crux of these observations is that if p53 is expressed in some way in cells having been in contact with biomaterials, this signals DNA damage (and possibly an initiation of cancer development).

This makes p53 an ideal candidate from among the many involved in cell cycle regulation.

Another such product is bcl-2 (from B-cell lymphoma). When overexpressed because of mutations, it will reduce p53 expression, thereby increasing the potential for cancer development. The expression of antiapoptotic proteins such as bcl-2 can inhibit apoptosis in response to many 'death-inducing' signals, and therefore demonstration of bcl-2 can also be used as a sign of mutation.

## 6.9  CONCLUSIONS

The following questions remain to be answered about the potential effect of apoptosis on biomaterials/biocompatibility evaluation:

- How can apoptosis be induced?
- Which methods to detect and measure apoptosis are relevant, practical and effective?
- Is apoptosis or oncosis (formerly necrosis) prevalent in cases of cytotoxicity of cells exposed to biomaterials or their extracts?
- Is there a correlation of apoptosis incidence with expression of proliferation markers or oncogene products?

Several methods are available to detect apoptosis, although many have been developed only recently. They have enormous potential for cytotoxicity testing of biomaterials and, possibly, for indirect detection of genetic aberrations.

One such method utilises the selective cutting of sites through DNA nick end-labelling (terminal deoxynucleotidyl transferase, TdT-mediated deoxyuridine, dUTP-biotin nick end-labelling, or TUNEL). It can be used on tissue sections as well as on cell cultures. Following exposure of DNA by proteolytic treatment, TdT is used to incorporate biotinylated dUTP at sites of DNA breaks. Avidin peroxidase can be used subsequently to amplify the signal, thereby allowing histology of the sections or cultures. The most important aspect of this treatment is the possibility of quantification.

A second method is the measurement of enrichment of mono- and oligonucleosomes in the cytoplasm before plasma membrane breakdown. After lysis of cells seeded on a 24-well plate, the cytoplasmic fractions are collected (centrifugation) and analysed in a sandwich ELISA assay, using monoclonal antihistone and anti-DNA antibodies, and a peroxidase detection system.

Agarose gel DNA electrophoresis (DNA ladder assay) or flow cytometry can also be used, apoptotic cells appearing as cells with a DNA content less than that of G1 cells.

## 6.10 REFERENCES

AS 2696(1984) Method of testing catheters for cytotoxicity. Philadelphia PA, USA.

ASTM F813-83(1983) standard practice for direct contact cell culture evaluation of materials for medical devices. ASTM, Philadelphia PA, USA.

ASTM F895-84 (1984) standard test method for agar diffusion cell culture screening for cytotoxicity. ASTM, Philadelphia PA, USA.

BS 5736(1988) Evaluation of medical devices for biological hazards, Part 10: Method of test for toxicity to cells in culture of extracts from medical devices. BSI, Milton Keynes, UK.

BS 5828(1989) Biological assessment of dental materials. BSI, Milton Keynes, UK.

DIN V13930(1990). Biologische prfungen von dentalwerkstoffen. DIN, Pforzheim, Germany.

FDA (1989) Guidance document for class III contact lenses. FDA, Rockville MD, USA.

Harmand MF, Bordenave L, Duphil R, Jeandot R and Ducassou D (1986) Human differentiated cell cultures: *in vitro* models for characterisation of the cell/biomaterial interface. In: Biological and biomechanical performances of biomaterials, Elsevier Science, 361–366.

ISO TR7405(1984) Biological evaluation of dental materials. ISO, Geneva, Switzerland.

Krammer PH, Behrmann I, Daniel P, Dhein J and Debatin KM (1994) Regulations of apoptosis in the immune system. Curr Opin Immunol 6:279-289.

Majno G and Joris F (1995) Review of apoptosis, oncosis and necrosis: An overview of cell death. Am J Pathol 146:3–15.

Naji A and Harmand MF(1991) Cytocompatibility of two coating materials, amorphous alumina and silicon carbide, using human differentiated cell cultures. Biomaterials 12:690–694.

NFS 90702 (1988a) Matériel médico-chirurgical: évaluation *in vitro* de la cytotoxicité des matériaux et dispositifs médicaux. Paris, France.

NFS 91-142 (1988b) Implants dentaires: cytocompatibilité – étude de la prolifération cellulaire. Paris, France.

NFS 91-143 (1988c) Implants dentaires: cytocompatibilité – étude des protéines cellulaires totales. Paris, France.

NFS 91-144 (1988d) Implants dentaires: évaluation du relargage extra-cellulaire du $^{51}$Cr. Paris, France.

NFS 91-145 (1988e) Implants dentaires: cytocompatibilité – étude de l'attachement et de l'étalement des cellules sur le biomatériau. Paris, France.

NFS 91-146 (1988f) Implants dentaires: cytocompatibilité – étude de la multiplication, la migration et l'adhésion cellulaire. Paris, France.

NFS 11-202 (1989a) Optique et instruments d'optique: cytocompatibilité des lentilles de contact – étude de la prolifération cellulaire. Paris, France.

NFS 11-203 (1989b) Optique et instruments d'optique: cytocompatibilité des lentilles de contact – évaluation des protéines cellulaires totales. Paris, France.

NFS 11-204 (1989c) Optique et instruments d'optique: cytocompatibilité des lentilles de contact – évaluation du relargage extracellulaire du $^{51}$Cr. Paris, France.

NFS 11-205 (1989d) Optique et instruments d'optique: cytocompatibilité des lentilles de contact – étude de l'attachement et de l'étalement des cellules sur le biomatériau. Paris, France.

NFS 11-206 (1989e) Optique et instruments d'optique: cytocompatibilité des lentilles de contact – étude de la multiplication, la migration et l'adhésion cellulaire. Paris, France.

PAB Notific. No.489 (1989) Approval standard of IOL in Japan. Tokyo, Japan.

USP (1990) The Pharmacopoeia of the USA. XXII, Biological reactivity tests *in vitro*.

Williams DF (ed.) (1991) Definitions in biomaterials. Proc. 2nd Consensus Conf. on Biomaterials, Chester, UK.

# 7
# Interactions with Blood

JAMES ANDERSON
Institute of Pathology, Case Western Reserve University, Cleveland, Ohio, USA

## 7.1 HISTORICAL PERSPECTIVE AND INTRODUCTION

The basis for this chapter is the ISO document 10993 Part 4: Selection of tests for interactions with blood. As indicated in Chapter 1, in the late 1980s ISO/TC 194 was convened to develop international harmonised standards dealing with the biological evaluation of medical devices (the 10993 series). Of the various WGs established, it was WG4 which was made responsible for addressing blood–material interactions through harmonisation of national standards and development of an international standard dealing with the selection of tests for interactions with blood.

This chapter utilises a similar outline to that provided by the ISO 10993-4 standard. However, it differs in that the normative and informative (annex) components of the standard have been intermixed to provide a more readable document, and components of ISO 10993-1: Guidance on selection of tests have been included to provide clarification and perspective.

In addition to the historical perspective and introduction section, this chapter has four additional sections:

• classification of categories of blood-contacting devices
• rationale and guidance for the structured selection of tests
• device-specific issues in the structured selection of tests
• perspectives on future standards modification and development with regard to tests for interactions with blood.

The purpose of ISO 10993-4 is to provide guidance to agencies, manufacturers, research laboratories and others for evaluating the interactions of medical devices with blood. The document describes a classification of medical and dental devices that are intended for use in contact with blood, based on the intended use and duration of contact as defined in ISO 10993-1. Furthermore, the document describes the fundamental principles governing the evaluation of the interaction of devices with blood and provides the rationale for the structured selection of tests, together with the principles and scientific bases of these tests. It should be

*Biocompatibility Assessment of Medical Devices and Materials.*
Edited by Julian Braybrook. © 1997 John Wiley & Sons Ltd.

noted that the standard states that the detailed requirements for testing cannot be specified because of the limitations in knowledge and precision of tests for interactions of devices with blood. These qualifying statements are deliberately included to obviate the possibility that users of the standard will not treat it simply as a checklist, but understand and provide a sound scientific rationale and justification for the selection of the tests for the unique material or device under consideration. Moreover, these qualifying tests acknowledge the possibility that new tests may become available which address specific blood component–material interactions, and which may be incorporated by users in their test protocol development. Regarding tests and test methods, investigators should refer to standard texts of laboratory medicine, haematology and clinical pathology (Miale, 1982; NIH, 1985; Corriveau and Fritsma, 1988; Kay, 1988; Dawids, 1993; Harker *et al.*, 1993; Colman *et al.*, 1994). The references for this chapter include references to scientific papers provided in ISO 10993-4 and those which will provide investigators with the additional rationale and scientific bases for carrying out tests to evaluate blood interactions with medical devices. References to the international and national standards provided in ISO 10993-4 are not included. Investigators should also refer to device-specific vertical standards for additional information on testing.

## 7.2  CLASSIFICATION OF CATEGORIES OF BLOOD-CONTACTING DEVICES

Historically, medical devices have been categorised by the nature and duration of their contact with the patient's body. Certain devices may fall into more than one category, in which case testing appropriate to each category should be considered. If a material or device may be placed in more than one duration category, the more rigorous testing requirements should apply. With multiple exposures, the decision into which category the device is placed should take into account the potential cumulative effect and time period over which these exposures occur.

### 7.2.1  NATURE OF CONTACT

'External communicating devices' and 'implant devices' are considered in the ISO 10993-4 standard, although non-contact devices (either directly or indirectly), i.e. *in vitro* diagnostic devices, are not.

External communicating devices are devices that contact the circulating blood and serve as a conduit into the vascular system. They are further categorised into bloodstream, indirect devices and circulating blood devices. The bloodstream and indirect devices contact the bloodstream at one point and serve as a conduit for entry into the vascular system. Examples include, but are not limited to:

- cannulae
- extension sets
- devices for the collection of blood
- devices for the storage and administration of blood
- blood products, e.g. tubing, needles and bags.

Such devices in contact with circulating blood include, but are not limited to:

- cardiopulmonary bypass systems
- extracorporeal membrane oxygenators
- haemodialysis equipment
- donor and therapeutic apheresis equipment
- devices for adsorption of specific substances from blood
- interventional cardiology and vascular devices
- percutaneous circulatory support systems
- temporary pacemaker leads and electrodes.

Implant devices are placed largely or entirely within the vascular system. Examples include, but again are not limited to:

- mechanical or tissue heart valves
- prosthetic or tissue vascular grafts
- circulatory support devices (ventricular assist devices (VADs), artificial hearts, intra-aortic balloon pumps)
- inferior vena cava (IVC) filters
- stents
- arteriovenous (AV) shunts
- blood monitors
- internal blood delivery catheters
- pacemaker leads and electrodes
- intravascular membrane oxygenators (artificial lungs).

These examples are given to aid investigators in identifying the nature of contact category to be considered for their unique device.

## 7.2.2  DURATION OF CONTACT

Three categories of exposure to blood have been identified for consideration by investigators when categorising their unique device by duration of contact. 'Limited exposure' is for devices whose single or multiple use or blood contact is likely to be up to 24 hours. 'Prolonged exposure' is for devices whose single, multiple or long-term use or blood contact is likely to exceed 24 hours, but not 30 days. 'Permanent contact' is for devices whose single, multiple or long-term use or blood contact exceeds 30 days. As indicated above, a material or device which may be used in more than one blood contact duration category should undergo the more rigorous testing requirements. If multiple exposure is likely,

**Table 7.1**   Blood–device interactions which may affect the device and its intended performance

| | |
|---|---|
| 1. | Adsorption of plasma proteins, lipids, calcium or other substances from the blood on to the surface of the device, or absorption of such substances into the device |
| 2. | Adhesion of platelets, leucocytes or erythrocytes on to the surface of the device, or absorption of their components into the device |
| 3. | Formation of pseudointima or tissue capsule on the surface of the device |
| 4. | Alterations in mechanical and other properties of the device |

**Table 7.2**   Blood–device interactions which may have an undesirable *in vivo* effect

Activation of platelets, leucocytes or other cells, or activation of the coagulation, fibrinolytic, complement or other pathways, including immunotoxicity (immunosuppression, immunopotentiation, immunomodulation)
Formation of thrombi on the device surface
Embolisation of thrombotic or other material from the device's luminal surface to another site within the circulation
Injury to circulating blood cells resulting in anaemia, haemolysis, leucopaenia, thrombocytopenia or altered function of blood cells
Injury to cells and tissues adjacent to the device
Intimal hyperplasia or accumulation of other tissue on or adjacent to the device, resulting in reduced flow or affecting other functions of the device
Adhesion and growth of bacteria or other infectious agents in or near the device

then the category of the material or device should take account of the potential cumulative effect, bearing in mind the period of time over which these exposures occur.

## 7.3   RATIONALE AND GUIDANCE FOR THE STRUCTURED SELECTION OF TESTS

### 7.3.1   GENERAL RECOMMENDATIONS AND CONSIDERATIONS

In addressing the development of a programme or protocol for the structured selection of tests, an understanding of blood–device interactions and their potential effects on the safety and efficacy of the *in vivo* performance of the device is critical.

Table 7.1 provides a list of interactions that may affect the device and which may or may not have an undesirable effect on performance. Test methods for the identification of these interactions should be considered for inclusion in the test method programme or protocol.

Table 7.2 presents interactions which may have a potentially undesirable effect

**Table 7.3** Device variables which may affect performance

| |
|---|
| The material(s) of manufacture |
| Intended additives, process contaminants and residues |
| Leachable substances |
| Degradation products |
| Other components and their interactions in the final product |
| The properties and characteristics of the final product |

on the subject (animal or human). In a similar fashion, test methods for identifying these interactions must be considered in the development of the test method protocol or programme.

The ISO 10993 standard stipulates biological evaluation of the medical device or biomaterial in its 'as used' state. This requirement indicates that the appropriate material processing conditions and method of sterilisation be carried out on materials, devices or parts or components of devices which will be in contact with blood. A material may be considered to be a medical device and includes any synthetic or natural polymer, metal, alloy, ceramic or other non-viable substance (including tissue rendered non-viable) which is used as a medical device or a part of a medical device.

In the selection of materials to be used in device manufacture the first consideration should be fitness for purpose, bearing in mind the characteristics and properties of the material, i.e. chemical, toxicological, physical, electrical, morphological and mechanical properties. Table 7.3 identifies other device variables which may affect performance. Investigators should have a good knowledge of the characteristics, properties and variables associated with the materials under consideration for utilisation in their respective devices.

In their structured selection, tests should use an appropriate model or system which simulates the geometry and conditions of contact of the device with blood during clinical applications (NIH, 1985; Harker *et al.*, 1993; Hanson *et al.*, 1980; Didisheim *et al.*, 1984a,b; Anderson and Kottke-Marchant, 1985; Cooper *et al.*, 1987; Dewanjee, 1987). These include duration of contact, temperature, sterility and flow. For devices of defined geometry, e.g. vascular grafts of varying lengths, the relation of surface area (length) to test results should be evaluated. Changes in design and/or flow conditions can alter the apparent *in vivo* haemocompatibility of a material: materials to be used in a low-flow (venous) environment may interact with blood differently when used in a high-flow (arterial) environment.

In the test protocol or programme, controls should be used unless their omission can be justified. Where possible, testing should include a device already in clinical use or well-characterised reference materials (RMs). The RMs used should include both negative and positive controls, bearing in mind animal welfare requirements. All materials tested should meet all quality control and quality assurance procedures of the manufacturer and test laboratory, and should be identified as to source, manufacture, grade and type.

**Table 7.4**    Criteria for re-evaluation of blood–device interactions

---

Any change in the source or specification of the materials used in the manufacture of the product

Any change in the formulation, processing, primary packaging or sterilisation of the product

Any change in the final product during storage

Any change in the intended use of the product

Any evidence that the product may produce adverse effects when used in humans

---

Bearing in mind the discussions outlined in Chapter 3 relating to 'worst case' and 'simulant' conditions, tests which do not simulate the conditions of a device during use may not accurately predict the nature of the blood–device interactions which may occur during clinical applications (Table 7.4).

For example, some short-term *in vitro* or *ex vivo* tests are poor predictors of long-term *in vivo* device interactions (Didisheim *et al.*, 1984a,b). The intended clinical application of the device should dictate the conditions under which it is tested, e.g. *ex vivo* (external communicating) devices should be tested *ex vivo*, and devices considered as implants should be tested *in vivo* in an animal model under similar conditions. If tests are selected in the manner described, the results have the greatest probability of predicting the clinical performance of devices. However, species differences and other factors may limit the predictability of any test, and thus human blood should be used where possible; where animal models are necessary, species differences in blood reactivity have to be considered (Didisheim *et al.*, 1984a,b; Cooper *et al.*, 1987; Dewanjee, 1987; Dewanjee *et al.*, 1992). The rationale and justification for the selection of a given species for *in vivo* testing should be provided in the test programme or protocol. Similarities and differences in blood cell and component reactivity between the chosen test species and humans should be provided. In blood–device testing, anticoagulants should be used only if the device is designed to perform in the presence of anticoagulants. The choice and concentration of anticoagulant used may influence blood–device interactions (Kottke-Marchant *et al.*, 1985) and so, if required, they should be used in the range of concentrations used clinically.

The test programme or protocol should include a sufficient number of tests, including suitable controls, to permit statistical evaluation of the resulting data. The variability in some test methods requires that they be repeated a sufficient number of times to determine significance. Repeated studies over an extended period of blood–device contact provide information about the time-dependent nature of the interactions. Again, animal welfare requirements should be borne in mind.

Circulating blood interacts with the luminal surfaces of medical devices under variable shear conditions to induce attachment of blood cells and plasma proteins, leading to variable:

- shear-dependent haemolysis
- activation of serine proteases comprising the complement, coagulation and fibrinolytic pathways
- secretion of granular contents of attached leucocytes and platelets
- thrombin-dependent platelet activation and fibrin production
- local formation of thrombi at sites in patterns that are flow dependent
- systemic embolisation of thrombotic material and/or thrombocellular aggregates.

As has been suggested, it is important to obtain objective measurements of blood–surface events as indicators of the relative importance of these phenomena and the potential usefulness of therapeutic interventions (Harker, 1994; Harker and Hanson, 1994).

## 7.3.2  TYPES OF TESTS

Three general types of tests are used to evaluate blood–device interactions: *in vitro*, *ex vivo* and *in vivo*. A combination of these is most commonly used. *In vitro* tests are commonly carried out for minutes to hours, *ex vivo* tests for hours to days, and *in vivo* tests for days to weeks to months. Care must be taken in the design and utilisation of a type of test to ensure that 'true' blood–device interactions are being measured and not artefacts of the type of test or test system.

### 7.3.2.1  *In vitro* Tests

Variables to be considered in the use of *in vitro* methods include haematocrit, anticoagulants, sample collection, sample age, aeration and pH, temperature, sequence of test vs control studies, surface-to-volume ratio, and fluid dynamic conditions (wall shear rate). Tests should be performed with minimal delay, as the properties of blood may change rapidly following collection. Both static and dynamic (flow) *in vitro* test systems should be considered, as there are significant differences between the two.

As *in vitro* systems most often utilise anticoagulants, human blood should be employed preferentially. Assays for human blood components are readily available and permit a comprehensive evaluation of blood–device interactions. Many of these assays are not available for animal blood components, and thus the predictability of tests utilising animal blood is limited. In some cases, the assays for human blood components may be utilised with non-human primate blood.

### 7.3.2.2  *Ex Vivo* Tests

*Ex vivo* tests permit the use of flowing native blood under appropriate physiological flow conditions and eliminate artefacts that may be caused by anticoagulants (Cooper *et al.*, 1987; Harker *et al.*, 1991; Zingg *et al.*, 1986). It is possible to monitor some blood–device interactions in real time. Such tests should be performed when the intended use of a device is *ex vivo*, e.g. an external communicating device. It may also be used when the intended use is *in vivo*, although this should not substitute for an implant test. *Ex vivo* test systems also allow blood flow rates to be measured, with variations indicating the extent and course of thrombus deposition and embolisation.

Disadvantages of *ex vivo* systems include variability in blood flow and reactivity between experiments and animal species respectively, and usually relatively short time intervals for evaluation purposes. Positive and negative controls using the same animal are recommended, bearing in mind animal welfare requirements.

### 7.3.2.3 *In Vivo* Tests

*In vivo* tests involve the implantation of the material or device in animals. As they usually involve the sacrifice of the animal following completion of the test, the opportunity for evaluation of thromboembolisation and infarction in organ systems is possible. Such tests should utilise the device in its 'as used' state.

In some *in vivo* test systems, the properties of the blood-contacting material may not be a major determinant of the blood–device interactions. Flow parameters, compliance, porosity and implant design may be more important than the blood compatibility of the material itself. With *in vivo* tests, it is important to recognise that a low flow-rate system may give substantially different results from a high flow-rate system.

The choice of an appropriate animal model for these tests may be restricted by size requirements, the availability of certain species and the cost. It is important that the investigators understand the physiological similarities and differences between the species chosen and those of the human. Data obtained from a single species should be interpreted with caution because of species differences in reactivity and variable responses to different devices.

Procedures to evaluate cardiovascular devices in animals are essentially the same as those employed in the human clinical setting. However, *in vivo* animal models permit continuous device monitoring and the systematic controlled study of important variables. It is important to appreciate that the surgical implant procedure may affect the results, and appropriate controls should be included.

### 7.3.3 *TEST METHODS: PRINCIPLES AND SCIENTIFIC BASIS*

The major modes of failure of cardiovascular devices and prostheses are thrombosis, thromboembolisation, bleeding and infection. To evaluate the mechanistic components of these failure modes, test methods to evaluate thrombosis, coagulation, platelets and platelet function, haematology and immunology are recommended. ISO 10993-4 provides recommended and optional tests for blood interactions with devices and materials. For the purposes of this chapter,

**Table 7.5** Recommended (Level 1) and optional (Level 2) tests for the interactions of external communicating devices and materials with blood

| Test category | Recommended method – Level 1, Bloodstream (indirect) | Recommended method – Level 1, circulating blood | Optional method – Level 2 |
|---|---|---|---|
| Thrombosis | Light microscopy (adhered platelets, leucocytes, aggregates, erythrocytes, fibrin, etc.) | % occlusion Flow reduction Gravimetric analysis (thrombus mass) Light microscopy (adhered platelets, leucocytes, aggregates, erythrocytes, fibrin etc.) Pressure drop across device | SEM (platelet adhesion and aggregation; platelet and leucocyte morphology; fibrin) |
| Coagulation | PTT (non-activated) | PTT (non-activated) | Specific coagulation factor assays FPA, D-dimer, $F_{1+2}$, PCA-1, S-12, TAT |
| Platelets | Platelet count | Platelet count Platelet aggregation Template bleeding time | PF-4, $\beta$-TG, thromboxane $B_2$ Gamma-imaging of radiolabelled platelets $^{111}$In-labelled platelet survival |
| Haematology | Leucocyte count and differential Haemolysis (plasma haemoglobin) | Leucocyte count and differential Haemolysis (plasma haemoglobin) | Reticulocyte count Activation specific release products of peripheral blood cells (i.e. granulocytes) |
| Immunology | C3a, C5a, TCC, Bb, iC3b, C4d, SC5b-9 | C3a, C5a, TCC, Bb, iC3b, C4d, SC5b-9 | IL-1 and other cytokines Detection of messenger-RNA specific for cytokines |

Table 7.5 (which gives the recommended Level 1 and optional Level 2 tests for the interactions of external communicating devices and materials with blood) is a compilation of the ISO 10993-4 Tables 2, 3 and 4.

Similarly Table 7.6, which presents recommended Level 1 and optional Level 2 tests for the interactions of implant devices and materials with blood, is a compilation of the ISO 10993-4 Tables 5 and 6 for implant devices.

For devices with limited blood exposure ( < 24 h), important measurements are related to the acute extent of variation of haematologic, haemodynamic and performance variables, gross thrombus formation and possible embolisation. With prolonged or repeated exposure, or permanent contact ( < 24 h), emphasis is placed on serial measurement techniques that may yield information regarding the time course of thrombosis and thromboembolisation, the consumption of

**Table 7.6** Recommended (Level 1) and optional (Level 2) tests for the interactions of implant devices and materials with blood

| Test Category | Recommended method – Level 1 | Optional method – Level 2 |
|---|---|---|
| Thrombosis | % occlusion<br>Flow reduction<br>Autopsy of device (gross and microscopic)<br>Autopsy of distal organs (gross and microscopic) | SEM<br>Angiography |
| Coagulation | PTT (non-activated), PT, TT<br>Plasma fibrinogen, FDP | Specific coagulation factor assays<br>FPA, D-dimer, $F_{1+2}$, PCA-1, S-12, TAT |
| Platelets | Platelet count<br>Platelet aggregation | [111]In-labelled platelet survival<br>PF-4, $\beta$-TG, thromboxane B2<br>Gamma-imaging of radiolabelled platelets |
| Haematology | Leucocyte count and differential<br>Haemolysis (plasma haemoglobin) | Reticulocyte count<br>Activation specific release products of peripheral blood cells (i.e. granulocytes) |
| Immunology | C3a, C5a, TCC, Bb, iC3b, C4d, SC5b-9 | IL-1 and other cytokines<br>Detection of messenger-RNA specific for cytokines |

circulating blood components, the development of intimal hyperplasia and infection. In both of the above exposure and contact categories, assessment of haemolysis is important. Thrombus formation may be greatly influenced by surgical technique, variable time-dependent thrombolytic and embolic phenomena, superimposed device infections and possible alterations in exposed surfaces (intimal hyperplasia and endothelialisation). The consequences of the interaction of artificial surfaces with blood may range from gross thrombosis and embolisation to subtle effects such as accelerated consumption of haemostatic elements, which may lead to depletion of platelets (thrombocytopenia) or plasma coagulation factors.

The recommended and optional test methods for the five test categories (thrombosis, coagulation, platelets and platelet function, haematology and immunology) were presented in Tables 7.5 and 7.6. It should be noted that common practice today is to include optional assays and test methods for the evaluation of blood–device interactions. This is in part due to the increased utilisation of human blood in *in vitro* dynamic (flow) tests.

### 7.3.3.1 Thrombosis

Test methods for thrombosis include percentage occlusion, flow reduction, gravimetric analysis (thrombus mass), light microscopy, scanning electron microscopy (SEM), pressure drop across the device, autopsy of the device, autopsy of distal organs and angiography (NIH, 1985; Schneider *et al.*, 1989; Colman, 1993; Dawids, 1993; Hanson, 1993).

Percentage occlusion is a measure of the severity of the thrombotic process in a conduit and is usually quantified after a device has been in use and then removed. Lack of occlusion does not necessarily eliminate the existence of a thrombotic process, as thrombi may have embolised or been dislodged before percentage occlusion is measured. Occlusion may be caused not only by thrombosis, but also by intimal hyperplasia (perianastomotic sites in vascular grafts or conduits), and microscopic examination is required to identify the nature of the occlusive process. Flow (rate or volume) may be measured over the course of the test. Gravimetric analysis of the thrombus mass may also be carried out following completion of the test and removal of the device. Light microscopy techniques or SEM evaluation may provide information regarding the density of cells, cellular aggregates and fibrin adherent to material and device surfaces, as well as the geographic distribution of these deposits on the surfaces. An opaque material may obviate light microscopy evaluation, and SEM is recommended under these circumstances. These methods are semiquantitative and quantitative conclusions require sufficient replicate determinations to establish reproducibility. Angiography is commonly used to determine the patency or degree of narrowing of a vascular graft or other conduit by detecting thrombus deposition on devices during their *in vivo* performance, and may provide correlation with alterations in flow rate or volume.

Following completion of the test, an autopsy of the device and distal organs of the animal (necropsy) may be carried out. The distribution, size and microscopic nature of cellular deposits can best be determined by a careful and detailed necropsy. Distal effects which may be observed include thromboembolism, infarction, infection and embolisation of the components of the device.

### 7.3.3.2 Coagulation Tests

Coagulation methods are based on the use of native (fresh, non-anticoagulated) whole blood, anticoagulated whole blood (usually citrated), platelet-rich plasma or platelet-poor plasma (Bithell, 1993; Boisclair *et al.*, 1993; Wachtfogel *et al.*, 1993). As most of the standard coagulation assays are designed to detect clinical coagulation disorders which result in delayed clotting or excessive bleeding, the protocols for evaluating blood–device interactions should be modified appropriately to evaluate accelerated coagulation induced by materials or devices.

The non-activated partial thromboplastin time (PTT) is recommended, as the activated PTT includes components which may mask the acceleration of coagulation induced by materials or devices; the material or device surface acts as the activating component in the non-activated assay and so controls should be included. Shortening of the PTT following contact with a material under standard conditions indicates activation of the contact phase of blood coagulation. A prolonged PTT suggests a deficiency in any of the coagulation factors I (fibrinogen), II (prothrombin), V, VIII, IX, X, XI or XII, but not VII or XIII. Heparin and other anticoagulants also cause a prolonged PTT. The prothrombin time (PT) and thrombin time (TT) are useful tests for the evaluation of implant devices only. A prolonged PT generally indicates a deficiency of prothrombin or factors V, VII, X or fibrinogen. The TT is prolonged with a deficiency in fibrinogen ($<100$ mg/dl), quantitative abnormalities in fibrinogen and elevated levels of fibrinogen degradation products (FDPs) or heparin. Alterations in fibrinogen, dysfibrogenaemia, afibrinogenaemia and hypofibrinogenaemia cause prolonged PT, PTT and TT results. The screening test most sensitive to fibrinogen deficiency is the TT. Exact levels of fibrinogen may be obtained with a commercially available modified PTT test. Fibrinogen and FDPs may be assayed for evaluating implant devices only. Immunoassay kits are available for fibrinogen and FDPs, but it is important to appreciate that these may be of no value when used with the blood of some animal species. Normally, low levels of FDPs are maintained by the low rate of the degradation reaction and the high rate of clearance of FDPs from the circulation. Pathological degradation of fibrin and fibrinogen, a result of increased plasminogen activation, yields FDP at levels $>2$ mg/ml.

Specific coagulation factor assays may show reduction of coagulation factors following exposure of blood to a material or device. Significant reduction of coagulation factors, e.g. to $<50\%$ of the normal or control level, suggest accelerated consumption of these factors by adsorption, coagulation or other mechanisms.

Activation of the coagulation mechanism may be evaluated by fibrinopeptide A (FPA), D-dimer fibrinogen or prothrombin F1 + 2 fragment measurements. Elevated thrombin–antithrombin complex (TAT) formation indicates activation of blood coagulation.

### 7.3.3.3 Platelets and Platelet Function

The evaluation of platelets, platelet function and platelet release products plays a significant role in the determination of blood–device interactions (Didisheim *et al.*, 1979; Harker *et al.*, 1980; Kottke-Marchant *et al.*, 1986; Dewanjee, 1987; Didisheim and Watson, 1990; Palatianos *et al.*, 1989; Hanson *et al.*, 1990; Dewanjee *et al.*, 1992; Malyszko *et al.*, 1995). Platelets play a key role in preventing bleeding and in thrombus formation. A significant drop in the platelet count of blood exposed to a device may be caused by platelet adhesion, platelet aggregation, platelet sequestration (e.g. in the spleen) or blood coagulation on the material surface. A reduction in platelet count during use of an implanted device may also be caused by accelerated destruction or removal of platelets from the circulation. Platelet concentrations may be determined manually or with the use of automated instruments. Platelet aggregation studies may reveal adverse blood–material interactions. Delayed or reduced platelet aggregation may be caused by platelet activation and the release of granular contents, increased FDP or certain drugs.

Blood cell adhesion is a measure of the blood compatibility of a material: the fewer blood cells that adhere, the more blood compatible is the material surface. Methods for blood cell adhesion assay may include direct counting of platelets, leucocytes etc., on the test surface or utilisation of a bead column. Alternatively, platelets prelabelled with $^{51}$Cr or $^{111}$In may be used.

The template bleeding time is an index of *in vivo* platelet function: a prolonged value suggests thrombocytopenia or a qualitative platelet disorder, such as may occur during cardiopulmonary bypass (Harker *et al.*, 1980).

Radionuclide imaging techniques using radiolabelled platelets may be used for the identification of thrombotic material on cardiovascular materials and devices (Cooper *et al.*, 1987; Dewanjee, 1987; Karwath *et al.*, 1989; Palatianos *et al.*, 1989; Hanson *et al.*, 1990; Dewanjee *et al.*, 1992). The gamma imaging of radiolabelled platelets may be carried out with platelets labelled with $^{111}$In, enabling the localisation and quantification of platelets deposited in a device. This method is useful for external communicating as well as implant devices.$^{111}$ In- (or $^{51}$Cr)-labelled platelets may also be utilised for platelet lifespan (survival) studies. Reduced platelet lifespan indicates accelerated removal from the circulation by immune, thrombotic or other processes. The utilisation of $^{111}$In labelling permits the assessment of localised platelet deposition with the lifespan (survival) study.

Platelet activation may be evaluated by the detection of different platelet membrane activation epitopes on circulating platelets and platelet microparticles using flow cytometry (Hanson *et al.*, 1988; Sheppeck *et al.*, 1991; Gemmell *et al.*, 1993; Cadroy *et al.*, 1994; Gemmell *et al.*, 1995; Kottke-Marchant *et al.*, 1995). This technique uses monoclonal antibodies (mAbs) which bind to the epitopes and, with the aid of a fluorescent dye, may be detected utilising flow cytometry, e.g. the use of PAC-1 (a mAb which recognises the activated form of platelet surface glycoprotein IIb/IIIa), S-12 (a mAb which recognises the α-granule membrane component GMP140, exposed during the platelet release reaction) and annexin V (a placental anticoagulant protein which detects aminophospholipid exposure and platelet membrane microparticle formation). Specific flow cytometric evaluation techniques will prove useful in the future in the detection of coagulation and platelet responses in blood–device interactions.

### 7.3.3.4  Haematology

Haemolysis is an especially significant screening test, as elevated plasma haemoglobin levels may indicate haemolysis and reflect red blood cell membrane fragility in contact with materials and devices. ISO 10993-4 recommends that a normative standard test method be used for the evaluation of haemolysis. Recently this test has come under scrutiny, as it appears that some investigators may have overinterpreted the results. It is important in carrying out this assay that appropriate controls be utilised to monitor plasma haemoglobin adsorption to the container surfaces, which would contribute to a false low plasma haemoglobin value.

Reticulocyte count measurements may indicate reduced red blood cell mass caused by chronic blood loss (bleeding), haemolysis or other mechanisms. An elevated reticulocyte count indicates increased production of red blood cells in the bone marrow.

Leucocyte counts and differential may indicate infection or adverse interactions with the material or device. An increased leucocyte count or shift in the differential distribution of leucocytes may suggest an infection.

### 7.3.3.5 Immunology

Elevated levels of C3a, C5a, TCC, Bb, iC3b, C4d and SC5b-9 complement components indicate activation of the complement system (Chenoweth and Henderson, 1987; Kottke-Marchant et al., 1987; Hakim, 1993; Cheung, 1994; Johnson, 1994; Rinder et al., 1995). These assays are important as activated complement components may activate leucocytes, enhancing their adhesion to material or device surfaces and/or causing them to aggregate and be sequestered in the lungs. Activation of leucocytes may lead to cytokine secretion, which may result in systemic and distal organ effects (Casey, 1993; Jahns et al., 1993; Dinarello, 1994). Cytokines play a major role in regulating the inflammatory and wound healing responses by controlling the growth of fibroblasts, smooth muscle cells and endothelial cells. Cytokines considered to be important at the present time are interleukin-1 (IL-1), IL-4, IL-6, tumour necrosis factor-$\alpha$ (TNF-$\alpha$), $\gamma$-interferon ($\gamma$-INF), and tissue growth factor-$\beta$ (TGF-$\beta$).

## 7.4  DEVICE-SPECIFIC ISSUES IN THE STRUCTURED SELECTION OF TESTS

As described in ISO 10993-1, the development of a structured programme of biological response tests focuses on the perspective that each device is unique, presents a unique set of characteristics, and thus may require a unique set of tests for biological response evaluation. With these perspectives in mind, the categorisation of tests is established on the basis of nature and duration of contact, and the intended application.

Thus this section presents issues, perspectives and comments on specific types of medical devices. The biological response evaluation may include both a study of relevant experience and actual testing. Such an evaluation may result in the conclusion that no testing is needed if the material has a demonstrable history of use in a specific role that is the same as the device under design. In addition, other information, including other non-clinical tests, clinical studies and postmarket experiences related to the device, may be included in the overall assessment programme. Common types of devices addressed in this section include cannulae, catheters and guidewires, extracorporeal oxygenators and similar devices, ventricular-assist devices, heart valve prostheses, vascular grafts, and inferior vena cava (IVC) filters and stents.

### 7.4.1 CANNULAE

Cannulae are typically inserted into one or more major blood vessels to provide repeated blood access. They may be used during cardiopulmonary bypass and other procedures, are tested acutely or chronically, and are commonly studied as AV shunts. The use of cannulae appears to induce little alteration in the levels of circulating blood cells or clotting factors (Lewis *et al.*, 1985). Cannulae, like other indirect bloodstream devices, generally require less testing than devices for circulating blood (see Table 7.5).

### 7.4.2 CATHETERS AND GUIDEWIRES

Most of the tests considered under cannulae are relevant to the study of catheters and guidewires. As the location or placement of catheters in the arterial or venous system can have a major effect on blood–device interactions, it is advised that simultaneous control studies be performed using a contralateral artery or vein. Care should be taken not to 'strip off' thrombi upon catheter removal. *In situ* evaluation may permit assessment of the extent to which intimal or entrance site injuries contribute to the thrombotic process. Kinetic studies with radiolabelled blood constituents are recommended only with chronic catheters, but may be useful for imaging thrombus accumulation *in vivo*. Angiography and Doppler blood flow measurements may also be useful.

### 7.4.3 EXTRACORPOREAL OXYGENATORS, HAEMODIALYSERS, THERAPEUTIC APHERESIS EQUIPMENT AND DEVICES FOR ABSORPTION OF SPECIFIC SUBSTANCES FROM BLOOD

The haemostatic response to cardiopulmonary bypass may be significant and acute. Many variables, e.g. use of blood suction, composition of blood pump priming fluid, hypothermia, blood contact with air and time of exposure, influence test results. Emboli in outflow lines may be detected by the periodic placement of blood filters *ex vivo* or the use of ultrasonic radiation or other non-invasive techniques. Thrombus accumulation can be directly assessed during bypass by monitoring performance factors, e.g. pressure drop across the oxygenator and oxygen transfer rate. An acquired transient platelet dysfunction associated with selected $\alpha$-granule release has been observed in some patients on cardiopulmonary bypass; the template bleeding time and other tests of platelet function and release are particularly useful in evaluating this phenomenon.

Complement activation is caused by both haemodialysers and cardiopulmonary bypass apparatus (Mahiout *et al.*, 1985; Spencer *et al.*, 1985; Borsch *et al.*, 1987;

Ward *et al.*, 1990). Clinically significant pulmonary leucostasis and lung injury with dysfunction may result, and for these reasons it is useful to quantify complement activation with these devices.

Therapeutic apheresis equipment and devices for absorption of specific substances from the blood, because of their high surface-to-volume ratio, can potentially activate complement, coagulation, platelet and leucocyte pathways. Examination of the blood–device interaction of these devices should follow the same principles as for extracorporeal oxygenators and hemodialysers.

## 7.4.4 *VENTRICULAR ASSIST DEVICES*

These devices may induce considerable alteration in various blood components. Factors contributing to such effects include the large foreign surface area to which blood is exposed, the high flow regimens and the regions of disturbed flow, e.g. turbulence or separated flow. Tests of such devices may include measurements of haemolysis, platelet and fibrinogen concentration, platelet survival, complement activation, and close monitoring of liver, renal, pulmonary and central nervous system function. Caution should be observed in interpreting test results as the surgical procedure itself may contribute extensively to changes in blood constituents. A detailed pathological examination at surgical retrieval is an important component of the evaluation (Burns *et al.*, 1987; Didisheim *et al.*, 1989; Schoen, 1989; Schoen *et al.*, 1990; Anderson, 1993; Schoen, 1995). Particular attention should be paid to the pathological evaluation of distal organs for the identification of thromboembolisation and infarction. The issues associated with explant retrieval and analysis are discussed in further detail in Chapter 10.

Harker has suggested that certain tests of blood interactions with artificial hearts be included in the structured test protocol, and these are listed in Table 7.7.

It is further suggested that these blood–surface interactions be monitored by performing measurements prior to implanting the artificial heart, and subsequently at the first week following implantation and each month thereafter. When artificial heart-bearing animals undergo autopsy, additional studies are suggested to evaluate prior thrombotic and thromboembolic events, namely:

- documentation of the location and extent of thrombus associated with the artificial heart and connecting segments
- morphometric analysis of infarcts in distal organs
- evaluation of isolated brains for the presence of cerebral infarction with selected validation by histology.

## 7.4.5 *HEART VALVE PROSTHESES*

Invasive, non-invasive and *in vitro* hydrodynamic studies are important in the assessment of prosthetic valves. Two D&M-mode echocardiography makes use of ultrasonic radiation to produce images of the heart: reflections from the materials

**Table 7.7** Suggested tests for the evaluation of blood interactions with artificial hearts

Complete blood cell counts (erythrocytes and reticulocytes, leucocytes with differential counts and platelets)
Plasma haemoglobin
Plasma TAT complex
$\beta$-TG
Binding of annexin V to platelets using flow cytometry
Ultrasonographic detection of microemboli in intracerebral and carotid arteries

with different acoustic impedances are received and processed to form an image. The structure of prosthetic valves can be examined. Mechanical prostheses emit strong echo signals and the movement of the occluder can usually be clearly imaged. However, the quality of the image may depend upon the particular valve being examined. Echocardiography may also be useful in the assessment of function of tissue-derived valve prostheses. Vegetations, clots and evidence of thickening of the valve leaflets are elucidated. Using conventional and colour-flow Doppler echocardiography, regurgitation can be identified and semiquantified.

Measurements of platelet survival and aggregation, blood tests of thrombosis and haemolysis, pressure and flow measurements, and autopsy of the valve and adjacent tissues are also recommended (Schoen, 1995). Plasma levels of the platelet-specific proteins PF-4 (platelet factor 4) and $\beta$-thromboglobulin ($\beta$-TG) may be useful in the evaluation of prosthetic heart valves.

## 7.4.6 VASCULAR GRAFTS

Both porous and non-porous materials can be implanted at various locations in the arterial or venous systems. The choice of implantation site is determined largely by the intended use of the prosthesis. The patency of a given graft is enhanced by a larger diameter and shorter length; a general rule for grafts less than 4 mm internal diameter is that the length should exceed the diameter by a factor of 10 (i.e. 40 mm for a 4 mm graft) for a valid model. Patency can be documented by palpation of distal pulses in some locations and by periodic angiography. Palpation of the vascular graft may lead to thrombosis, and caution should be observed in utilising this technique. Ultrasonic radiation, MRI (magnetic resonance imaging) and PET (positron emission tomography) may also be useful. Results of serial radiolabelled platelet imaging studies correlate with the area of non-endothelialised graft surface in baboons. Radiolabelled platelets facilitate non-invasive imaging of mural thrombotic accumulations. Serial measurements of platelets, platelet release constituents, fibrinogen/FDPs and activated coagulation species are also recommended. Autopsy of the graft and adjacent vascular segments for morphometric studies of endothelial integrity and healing responses can provide valuable information (Anderson, 1993).

## 7.4.7   IVC FILTERS AND STENTS

These devices can be studied by angiography and ultrasonic radiation. Other techniques useful for vascular graft evaluation are also appropriate for evaluation of these devices.

Vascular interventional devices are commonly used to treat atherosclerotic disease. Thus, an animal model, i.e. rabbit or pig, in which atherosclerosis and the formation of atherosclerotic plaques are induced, is generally recommended for these studies. Of particular importance in these animal studies is the histological evaluation of the healing response as it relates to restenosis.

## 7.5   PERSPECTIVES ON FUTURE STANDARDS MODIFICATION AND DEVELOPMENT

In considering the modification and development of future standards, it must be remembered that standards development is an iterative process which must constantly undergo revision as the state of the art technology pertinent to a specific standard evolves. Furthermore, ISO 10993 was designed and developed to be a horizontal standard and not a product-specific vertical one. Thus, for the future, it may be helpful to review the past in regard to the ideas and concepts under which ISO 10993 was developed.

First, each material or device is considered to have unique characteristics which require a unique programme of evaluation for biocompatibility or biological response. This perspective is incorporated in the ISO 10993-1 document, which states: 'due to the diversity of medical devices, it is recognised that not all tests identified in a category will be necessary or practical for any given device. It is indispensable for testing that each device shall be considered on its own merits: additional tests not indicated in the table may be necessary'. This forces the investigator to play an active role in the test method protocol or programme design and development. Of course, this statement also requires that appropriate rationale and justification be provided for the inclusion or omission of test methods based on the unique characteristics of the material or device under consideration.

These concepts and perspectives will be more significant and important in the future as new materials and devices designed for deliberate and specific interactions with blood components are developed and utilised. An example of this is heparinised surfaces, which are currently being developed and used clinically. As devices, special emphasis is placed on test methods which examine the coagulation system and the role played by surface-bound heparin in modulating the coagulation system at the interface (Elgue et al., 1993; Boonstra et al., 1994; Pekna et al., 1994; Kirschfink et al., 1993; Ernofsson et al., 1995; Kottke-Marchant et al., 1995; Mollnes et al., 1995; Sanchez et al., 1995). A second example is the covalent binding of adhesion ligands to surfaces for the attachment of cells (Hubbell, 1993; Schoen *et al.*, 1993; NIH, 1995). In regard to the biological response testing of these types of surfaces, test methods directed toward evaluating the cell function and phenotypic expression of attached cells must be utilised in the biological response evaluation.

As already indicated in the previous chapters, ISO 10993 was not intended to be a set of definitive statements, a checklist for investigators or regulators. It was designed and developed to be applied with interpretation and judgement by appropriate professionals qualified by training and experience.

The science of today will result not only in the materials and devices of tomorrow but also in the test methods by which these new materials and devices will be evaluated for their biological responses. Tissue engineering is an emerging discipline that applies engineering principles to create devices for the study, restoration, modification and assembly of functional tissues and organs from native or synthetic sources (NIH, 1995). As this discipline develops and incorporates new knowledge and information regarding:

- biological signals and signal mechanisms in cardiovascular devices
- normal and directed healing mechanisms in cardiovascular devices
- delivery and phenotypic expression of cells in and on cardiovascular devices

the knowledge base developed will also provide the test methods by which these devices will be evaluated, and which will be incorporated into standards designed to address issues of biocompatibility, safety and efficacy.

In the future development of new standards which address the selection of tests for interactions with blood, it is important that we continue to emphasise the complex and interactive milieu of the cellular and humoral components that constitute blood. We must continue to appreciate the interactive environment provided by the numerous humoral enzyme systems (kinin, fibrinolytic, coagulation and complement), formed elements (platelets), and cells (polymorphonuclear leucocytes, monocytes, lymphocytes and eosinophils) which provide for positive (activating) and negative (inhibiting) interactions. Failure to appreciate these types of interactions and feedback control mechanisms may lead to false interpretation of results from single or isolated test methods. An example might be the use of an immunoassay for the quantitative determination of IL-1 (Bonfield *et al.*, 1992; Bonfield and Anderson, 1993; Dinarello, 1994). High plasma levels of IL-1, with its known cellular and systemic effects, may lead an investigator towards one interpretation, although such levels may not be reflective of biological activity, as the IL-1 receptor antagonist (IL-1ra) is known to inhibit the effect of IL-1 and downregulate or inhibit the biological effects of IL-1. Thus, it is possible, through feedback and inhibitory mechanisms, to downregulate biological responses. A broader perspective must be taken in the future regarding selection of tests for interactions with blood as it relates to the quantitative determination of parameters vs the biological response evaluation of parameters.

As our knowledge base for the research and development of new cardiovascular materials increases, enhanced integration of disciplines affecting test methods and standards development will be necessary. This will increase the dependence of regulatory agencies and bodies on the scientific community for test method development and interpretation. Hopefully, this will in turn lead to the development of a partnership between those who develop and test cardiovascular materials and devices, and those who are responsible for their regulation. Regardless of one's perspective, the overall goal is the assurance of safety and efficacy of cardiovascular devices for clinical use.

## 7.6 REFERENCES

Anderson JM (1993) Cardiovascular device retrieval and evaluation. Cardiovasc Pathol 2(3):199S–208S.

Anderson JM and Kottke-Marchant K (1985) Platelet interactions with biomaterials and artificial devices. CRC Crit Rev Biocompat 1(2):111–204.

Bithell TC (1993) Blood coagulation. In: Lee GR, Bithell TC, Foerster J, Athens JW and Lukens JN (eds.) Wintrobe's Clinical Haematology. Lea and Febiger, Philadelphia PA, USA, pp. 566–615.

Boisclair MD, Lane DA, Philippou H et al. (1993) Mechanisms of thrombin generation during surgery and cardiopulmonary bypass. Blood 82:3350–3357.

Bonfield TL and Anderson JM (1993) Functional vs quantitative comparison of IL-1b from monocytes/macrophages on biomedical polymers. J Biomed Mater Res 27:1195–1199.

Boonstra PW, Gu YJ, Akkerman C et al. (1994) Heparin coating of an extracorporeal circuit partly improves haemostasis after cardiopulmonary bypass. J Thorac Cardiovasc Surg 107:289–292.

Borsch T, Schmidt B, Blumenstein M and Gurland HJ (1987) Thrombogenicity markers in clinical and ex vivo assessment of membrane biocompatibility. Contr Nephrol 59:90–98.

Burns GL, Pantalos GM and Olsen DB (1987) The calf as a model for thromboembolic events with the total artificial heart. Trans Am Soc Artif Int Organs 33:398–403.

Cadroy Y, Hanson SR, Kelly AB et al. (1994) Relative antithrombotic effects of mAbs targeting different platelet glycoprotein–adhesive molecule interactions in non-human primates. Blood 83(11):3218–3224.

Casey LC (1993) Role of cytokines in the pathogenesis of cardiopulmonary-induced multisystem organ failure. Ann Thorac Surg 56:S92–S96.

Chenoweth DE and Henderson LW (1987) Complement activation during haemodialysis: Laboratory evaluation of haemodialysers. Artif Organs 11:155–162.

Cheung AK (1994) Complement activation as index of haemodialysis membrane biocompatibility: the choice of methods and assays. Nephrol Dial Transplant 9(2)S:96–103.

Colman RW (1993) Mechanism of thrombus formation and dissolution. Cardiovasc Pathol 2:23S–31S.

Colman RW, Hirsh J, Marder VJ and Salzman EW (eds.) (1994) Haemostasis and thrombosis: basic principles and clinical practice, 3rd edn. Lippincott, Philadelphia PA, USA.

Cooper SL, Fabrizius DJ and Grasel TG (1987) Methods of assessment of thrombosis ex vivo. Ann NY Acad Sci 516:572–585.

Corriveau DM and Fritsma GA (eds) (1988) Haemostasis and thrombosis in the clinical laboratory, Lippincott, Philadelphia PA, USA.

Dawids S (ed.) (1993) Test procedures for the blood compatibility of biomaterials. Kluwer Academic Publishers, Dordrecht, The Netherlands.

Dewanjee MK (1987) Methods of assessment of thrombosis *in vivo*. Ann NY Acad Sci 516:541–571.

Dewanjee MK, Kapadvanjwala M and Sanchez A (1992) Quantitation of comparative thrombogenicity of dog, pig and human platelets in a haemodialyser. Am Soc Artif Int Organs J 38:88–90.

Didisheim P, Stropp JQ, Borowick JH and Grabowski EF (1979) Species differences in platelet adhesion to biomaterials: Investigation by a two-stage technique. Trans Am Soc Artif Int Organs 2:124–132.

Didisheim P, Dewanjee MK, Frisk CS, Kaye MP and Fass DN (1984a) Animal models for predicting clinical performance of biomaterials for cardiovascular use. In: Boretos JW and Eden M (eds.) Contemporary biomaterials. Noyes, Park Ridge NJ, USA, pp. 132–179.

Didisheim P, Dewanjee MK, Kaye MP et al. (1984b) Non-predictability of long-term *in vivo* response from short-term *in vitro* or *ex vivo* blood/material interactions. Trans Am Soc Artif Int Organs 30:370–376.

Didisheim P and Watson JT (1989) Thromboembolic complications of prosthetic devices and artificial surfaces. In: Kwaan HC and Samama MM (eds) Clinical thrombosis. CRC Press, Boca Raton FL, USA.

Didisheim P, Olsen DB, Farrar DJ et al. (1989) Infections and thromboembolism with implantable cardiovascular devices. Trans Am Soc Artif Int Organs 35:54–70.

Dinarello CA (1994) The IL-1 family: 10 years of discovery. FASEB J 8:1314–1325.

Elgue G, Sanchez J, Egberg N, Olsson P and Riesenfeld J (1993) Effect of surface-immobilised heparin on the activation of adsorbed factor XII. Artif Organs 17:721–726.

Ernofsson M, Thelin S and Siegbahn A (1995) Thrombin generation during cardiopulmonary bypass using heparin-coated circuits or conventional circuits. Thromb Haemost 73:1344.

Gemmell CH, Sefton MV and Yeo EL (1993) Platelet-derived microparticle formation involves GPIIb/IIIa: inhibition by RGDS and a Glanzmann's thrombasthenia defect. J Biol Chem 268:14586–14589.

Gemmell CH, Ramirez SM, Yeo EL and Sefton MV (1995) Platelet activation in whole blood by artificial surfaces: Identification of platelet-derived microparticles and activated platelet binding to leucocytes as material-induced activation events. J Lab Clin Med 125:276–287.

Hakim RM (1993) Complement activation by biomaterials. Cardiovasc Pathol 2:187S–197S.

Hanson SR (1993) Device thrombosis and thromboembolism. Cardiovasc Pathol 2:157S–165S.

Hanson SR, Harker LA, Ratner BD and Hoffman AS (1980) *In vivo* evaluation of artificial surfaces using a non-human primate model of arterial thrombosis. J Lab Clin Med 95:289–304.

Hanson SR, Pareti FI, Ruggeri ZM (1988) Effects of mAbs against the platelet glycoprotein IIb/IIIa complex on thrombosis and haemostasis in the baboon. J Clin Invest 81:149–158.

Hanson SR, Kotze HF, Pieters H and Heyns A duP (1990) Analysis of [111]In platelet kinetics and imaging in patients with aortic aneurysms and abdominal aortic grafts. Arteriosclerosis 10:1037–1044.

Harker LA (1994) New antithrombotic strategies for resistant thrombotic processes. J Clin Pharmacol 34:3–16.

Harker LA and Hanson SR (1994) Platelet factors predisposing to arterial thrombosis. Bailliere's Clinical Haematology 7(3):499–522.

Harker LA, Malpass TW, Branson HE, Hessel EA and Slichter SJ (1980) Mechanism of abnormal bleeding in patients undergoing cardiopulmonary bypass: Acquired transient platelet dysfunction associated with selective alpha granule release. Blood 56:824–834.

Harker LA, Kelly AB and Hanson SR (1991) Experimental arterial thrombosis in non-human primates. Circulation 83(IV):41–55.

Harker LA, Ratner BD and Didisheim P (eds.) (1993) Cardiovascular biomaterials and biocompatibility. Supplement to Cardiovascular Pathology. Elsevier, NY, USA.

Hubbell JA (1993) Pharmacologic modification of materials. Cardiovasc Pathol 2:121S–127S.

Jahns G, Haeffner-Cavaillon N, Nydegger UE and Kazatchkine MD (1993) Complement activation and cytokine production as consequences of immunological bioincompatibility of extracorporeal circuits. Clin Mater 14:303–336.

Johnson RJ (1994) Complement activation during extracorporeal therapy: biochemistry, cell biology and clinical relevance. Nephrol Dial Transplant 9(2)S:36–45.

Karwath R, Schürer M and Wolf H (1989) Measurement of platelet adhesiveness on to artificial surfaces using $^{51}$Cr and $^{111}$In-labelled platelets. Studia Biophysica 131:117–123.

Kay LA (1988) Essentials of haemostasis and thrombosis. Churchill Livingstone, Edinburgh, UK.

Kirschfink M, Kovacs B and Mottaghy K (1993) Extracorporeal circulation: *in vivo* and *in vitro* analysis of complement activation by heparin-bonded surfaces. Circulatory Shock 40:221–226.

Kottke-Marchant K, Anderson JM, Rabinovitch A, Huskey RA and Herzig R (1985) The effect of heparin *vs* citrate on the interaction of platelets with vascular graft materials. Thromb Haemost 54:842.

Kottke-Marchant K, Anderson JM and Rabinovitch A (1986) The platelet reactivity of vascular graft prostheses: an *in vitro* model to test the effect of preclotting. Biomaterials 7:441–448.

Kottke-Marchant K, Anderson JM, Miller KM, Marchant RE and Lazarus H (1987) Vascular graft-associated complement activation and leucocyte adhesion in an artificial circulation. J Biomed Mater Res 21:379–397.

Kottke-Marchant K, Borsch J, McCarthy P et al. (1995) Platelet and coagulation activation by heparin-coated cardiopulmonary bypass systems. Thromb Haemost 73:1344.

Lewis JL, Sweeney J, Baldini L, Friedland GH and Salzman EW (1985) Assessment of thromboresistance of intravenous cannulae by $^{125}$I-fibrinogen scanning. J Biomed Mater Res 19:99.

Mahiout A, Meinhold H, Jorres A et al. (1985) *Ex vivo* model for preclinical evaluation of dialysers containing new membranes. Life Support Systems 3(S1):448–452.

Malyszko J, Malyszko JS, Borawski J et al. (1995) A study of platelet functions, some haemostatic and fibrinolytic parameters in relation to serotonin in haemodialysed patients under erythropoietin therapy. Thromb Haemost 77:133–143.

Miale JB (1982) Laboratory medicine haematology, 6th edn. Mosby CV, St. Louis MO, USA.

Mollnes TE, Riesenfeld J, Garred P et al. (1995) A new model for evaluation of biocompatibility: Combined determination of neo-epitopes in blood and on artificial surfaces demonstrates reduced complement activation by immobilisation of heparin. Artif Organs 19(9):909–917.

NIH (1985) Guidelines for blood/material interactions. Report of the NHLBI WG, US Dept. of Health and Human Services, NIH, Publ. No.85-2185.

NIH (1995) Tissue engineering in cardiovascular disease: a report. J Biomed Mater Res 29:1473–1475.

Palatianos GM, Dewanjee MK and Robinson RP (1989) Quantitation of platelet loss with $^{111}$In-labelled platelets in a hollow-fiber membrane oxygenator and arterial filter during extracorporeal circulation in a pig model. Trans Am Soc Artif Int Organs 35:667–670.

Pekna M, Hagman L, Halden E et al. (1994) Complement activation during cardiopulmonary bypass: Effects of immobilised heparin. Ann Thorac Surg 58:421–424.

Rinder CS, Rinder HM, Smith BR et al. (1995) Blockade of C5a and C5b-9 generation inhibits leucocyte and platelet activation during extracorporeal circulation. J Clin Invest 96:1564–1572.

Sanchez J, Elgue G, Riesenfeld J and Olsson P (1995) Control of contact activation on end-point immobilised heparin: the role of antithrombin and the specific antithrombin-binding sequence. J Biomed Mater Res 29:655–661.

Schneider PA, Kotze HF, Heyns A duP and Hanson SR (1989) Thromboembolic potential of synthetic vascular grafts in baboons. J Vasc Surg 10:75–82.

Schoen FJ (1989) Interventional and surgical pathology – Appendix: Pathologic analysis of the cardiovascular system and prosthetic devices. WB Saunders, Philadelphia PA, USA.

Schoen FJ (1995) Approach to the analysis of cardiac valve prostheses as surgical pathology or autopsy specimens. Cardiovasc Pathol 4:241–255.

Schoen FJ, Anderson JM, Didisheim P et al. (1990) VAD pathology analyses: guidelines for clinical studies. J Appl Mater 1:49–56.

Schoen FJ, Libby P and Didisheim P (1993) Future directions and therapeutic approaches. Cardiovasc Pathol 2(3):209S–216S.

Sheppeck RA, Bentz M, Dickson C (1991) Examination of the roles of GPIb and GPIIb/IIIa in platelet deposition on artificial surfaces using clinical antiplatelet agents and mAb blockade. Blood 78:673–680.

Spencer PC, Schmidt B, Samtleben W, Bosch T and Gurland HJ (1985) Ex vivo model of haemodialysis membrane biocompatibility. Trans Am Soc Artif Int Organs 31:495–498.

Wachtfogel YT, dela Cadena RA and Colman RW (1993) Structural biology, cellular interactions and pathophysiology of the contact system. Thromb Res 72:1–21.

Ward RA, Schmidt B, Blumenstein M and Gurland HJ (1990) Evaluation of phagocytic cell function in an ex vivo model of hemodialysis. Kidney Int 37:776–782.

Zingg W, Ip WF, Sefton MV and Mancer K (1986) A chronic AV shunt for the testing of biomaterials and devices in dogs. Life Support Systems 4:221–229.

# 8
# Genotoxicity, Carcinogenicity and Reproductive Toxicity

ROSY ELOY AND N. WEILL
Biomatech, Chasse-sur-Rhône, France

## 8.1  INTRODUCTION

Although biomaterials have long been considered as inert, non-biologically interacting materials, it is now recognised that their interaction with cell cycle regulation should be evaluated critically. The associated risk may be related to one or more of the following factors at the site of implantation of a medical device:

- leaching of one critical component, e.g. ion, chemical, polymer, additive, plasticiser etc.
- surgical, thermal or mechanical injury at the time of implantation
- degradation products interacting with the normal cell metabolism
- the nature of the interface, shape, porosity, pore size and roughness.

Compared to other risks covered by the different standards for evaluating biocompatibility, the methods for assessment of genotoxicity, carcinogenicity or reproductive toxicity are neither equally well developed nor is their validity for testing medical devices well established. One important characteristic of these risks is also the latency for their development, which implies that predictive models dealing with this parameter need to be developed.

It is also important to be fully conversant with the definitions for each of the topics considered here. A substance is considered to be:

- carcinogenic, if it can be shown to be related causally to an increased incidence of malignant neoplastic formation
- mutagenic, if it induces alteration in the genetic code of the cell
- tumorigenic, if it can be shown to be related causally to an increased incidence of neoplastic formation, whether malignant or benign.

Mechanistically, a mutagenic product generally has to induce a primary lesion of DNA. This lesion will usually be repaired by DNA repair enzymes, but if these systems are deficient, non-existent or overworked, the lesion will persist in the

*Biocompatibility Assessment of Medical Devices and Materials.*
Edited by Julian Braybrook. © 1997 John Wiley & Sons Ltd.

DNA and, when the cell divides, may be transformed into a mutation. Cells exhibiting too large a number of DNA lesions will tend to die, either directly or by apoptosis (considered earlier in Chapter 6), whereas those exhibiting fewer lesions will tend to remain viable.

The relevant ISO-10993 standard which deals specifically with these topics, Part 3 (ISO, 1994) provides definitions for the following associated tests:

- genotoxicity test – a test that applies mammalian or non-mammalian cells, bacteria, yeasts or fungi to determine whether gene mutations, changes in chromosome structure, or other DNA or gene changes are caused by the test materials, devices and/or extracts from materials. Tests on whole animals may also address these end-points.
- carcinogenicity test – a test to determine the tumorigenic potential of devices, materials and/or extracts to either a single or multiple exposures over a period of the total life-span of the test animal. These tests may be designed to examine both chronic toxicity and tumorigenicity in a single experimental study.
- reproductive and developmental toxicity tests – tests to evaluate the potential effects of devices, materials and/or extracts on reproductive function, embryonic development (teratogenicity), and prenatal and early postnatal development.

Each of these topics will now be considered in further detail.


## 8.2  MUTAGENICITY

### 8.2.1  GENERAL CONSIDERATIONS (Forster, 1986)

Mutation is an inheritable genetic change. Two main classes of mutations are recognised:

- mutations in individual genes, involving changes in the sequence of bases in DNA or frame shift mutations which alter the coding
- chromosomal mutations, involving alterations to the number of chromosomes or chromosome structure anomalies.

A mutagen is an agent that increases the rate at which these mutations occur, although it should be recognised that mutations also occur spontaneously at a very low rate. Thus investigation of the mutagenic effect of a chemical should take account of the ability to cause gene mutation, alter chromosomal structure or numbers or damage DNA. A panel of mutagenicity tests is given in Table 8.1.

*In vitro* test systems may be divided into those employing prokaryotic and those employing eukaryotic test organisms. The genetic apparatus of prokaryotic organisms is helpfully simple, since genes are generally present in one copy only, on a single circular chromosome. However, eukaryotic organisms have a chromosomal organisation and genes may be present in more than one copy on homologous chromosomes.

**Table 8.1**   Classification of selected, well-known mutagenicity tests

| | |
|---|---|
| Tests for gene mutation | |
| *In vitro* | Ames test or *E.coli* test |
| | Gene mutation in cultured mammalian cells |
| | Sex-linked recessive lethal test (*Drosophila*) |
| *In vivo* | Mouse coat-colour 'spot test' |
| | |
| Tests for chromosomal damage | |
| *In vitro* | Mitotic aneuploidy in yeast |
| | Metaphase analysis of cultured mammalian cells |
| *In vivo* | Micronucleus test |
| | Metaphase analysis of treated animal |
| | |
| Test for DNA damage | |
| *In vitro* | Mitotic gene conversion in yeast |
| | Sister chromatid exchange |
| | Unscheduled DNA synthesis |
| | Alkaline elution assay |
| | SOS induction tests |
| | Differential killing assays |

Some of these tests are also designed to detect mutations in somatic cells (e.g. the mouse spot test), whereas others detect mutations in germ cells. In addition, during the 1950s it became apparent that foreign-body compound metabolism played an important role in chemical carcinogenesis by converting some chemicals into reactive electrophilic forms able to react with proteins and nucleic acids. Metabolising systems therefore became a standard for most *in vitro* mutagenicity assays.

Assay methods must take into account two kinds of mutagens:

- the reactive chemical which can damage DNA directly without any metabolic step
- those chemicals which are mutagenic only after conversion to reactive intermediates by metabolic activation.

Both gene mutation and chromosomal effects studies are mandatory according to ISO 10993-3, which also recommends the inclusion of at least one *in vivo* investigation in a mammalian organism. In addition, the effects of product degradation *in vivo* and/or the effects of product metabolism should be evaluated in an *in vivo* model evaluating the mutagenic effects in the conditions of use.

## 8.2.2   ASSAYS FOR POINT MUTATION: MICROBIAL

### 8.2.2.1   Ames Test

This test is based on the use of five specifically constructed strains of *Salmonella typhimurium* containing a specific mutation in the histidine operon and other mutations that increase their ability to detect mutagens (Ames *et al.*, 1975). These genetically altered strains cannot grow in the absence of histidine. When they are placed in a histidine-free medium, only those cells which mutate spontaneously back to the wild type (non-histidine dependent by way of manufacture of their own histidine) are able to form colonies. The spontaneous mutation rate (or reversion rate) for any one strain is relatively constant, but if a mutagen is added to the system the mutation rate is significantly increased. Metabolic activation is achieved by the use of liver homogenates from rats stimulated with Aroclor 1254 or a mixture of phenobarbital and methylcholanthrene.

An extraction vehicle without test material is used with each test strain to determine the spontaneous reversion rate, and represents the negative control. Known mutagens are used as positive controls.

A preliminary toxicity screen is carried out and evaluated to determine whether dilution of the extract is not inhibitory to the test strains.

The test article extract, negative control and the different mutagens are all tested, in triplicate, with and without metabolic activation. Following the incubation period, spontaneous revertants from each plate are recorded and the mean number compared for each of the five test strains employed (TA 98-100, TA 1535, TA 1537 and TA 1538 or TA 102) to that with the negative control. Potential mutagens induce a twofold or greater increase in the number of mean revertants over the values obtained for the negative control.

### 8.2.2.2   *E. Coli* Test

This test is based upon the use of *Escherichia coli* strain WP2 containing specific mutations in the tryptophan operon. These strains could be used in addition to, or in place of, the *Salmonella* strains described above.

### 8.2.2.3   Mouse Lymphoma Test

In this test, cells that have the enzyme thymidine kinase (TK) are sensitive to the toxic action of trifluorothymidine (TFT), which is metabolised in a false metabolite incorporated in the nucleic acids. The cells that exhibit the mutated TK gene cannot form the false metabolite and survive in the presence of TFT.

### 8.2.3   *TESTS FOR CHROMOSOMAL DAMAGE*

These tests provide evidence of the induction of anomalies to the chromosome structure and, to a lesser extent, the number of affected chromosomes. A clastogenic product is one able to induce chromosome breaks.

Structural damage to chromosomes may include exchanges of materials between chromosomes or chromatids, deletions, breaks and all the aberrations resulting from these events. Chromosomes are also encountered that are completely fragmented (shattered) by exposure to test chemicals. Numerical changes commonly include the loss or gain of chromosomes to produce aneuploid cells, or the presence of multiple copies of the genome (polyploidy).

To perform an *in vitro* assay for chromosomal damage the following procedure is used. Cultures of mammalian cells are treated with the test chemical, in both the presence and the absence of S9 metabolism. The cell type employed for the assay is a matter of choice: human lymphocytes offer a convenient source of human material, although Chinese hamster cells are often employed because they are robust, have a relatively small number of chromosomes and the scorer can soon become familiar with the karyotype. The chromosomes are most clearly observed in cells which are in the metaphase stage of mitosis and, in order to increase the yield of cells in this phase, the spindle poison colchicine is frequently used. Colchicine is added to the cultures during the latter part of the treatment period, and finally the cells are harvested and prepared for microscope slide observation. Chromosomal damage is assessed by inspecting a large number of metaphases from the control and treated populations. Any aberrant structures are interpreted and classified, e.g. a break may affect either one or both of the chromatids of a chromosome, and thus be classified as a chromatid or chromosome break (Figure 8.1).

This kind of assay can readily be performed in whole animals and it is only necessary to treat groups of laboratory animals and, at sacrifice, to harvest cells from proliferating tissue: bone marrow cells are commonly used.

In addition, however, a rapid and convenient method for assessing chromosome damage *in vivo* is offered by the micronucleus test. This assay depends upon the fact that chromosome fragments fail to align normally in the later stages of cell division and are excluded from the nuclei in that form; instead, they form small secondary nuclei, called micronuclei. These are readily recognisable and easy to score (Figure 8.2). They are rare in normal dividing cells, but their incidence is increased by treatment with known clastogens.

The developing erythrocytes of mice offer a convenient system to study micronuclei, as the erythrocytes do not expel the micronuclei when they enucleate. Young erythrocytes which have recently divided are the most appropriate cells to examine because:

• they retain some ribosomal RNA in their cytoplasm
• they can be distinguished from mature erythrocytes by differential staining: the young cells (polychromatid erythrocytes, PCEs) stain pale blue, whereas the mature cells (normochromatid erythrocytes, NCEs) stain pink.

The bone marrow is a rich source of PCEs. Thus, to perform a micronucleus test, groups of animals are treated with the test extract or implanted with the material to be tested and, after an appropriate treatment period, are sacrificed; the femoral bone marrow is recovered and smear slides are prepared and stained differentially. About 1000 PCEs from each animal are then scored for micronuclei. The micronucleus incidence in the treatment groups is compared with concurrent vehicle controls.

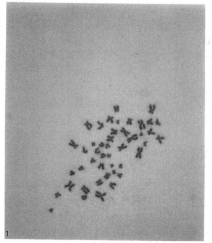
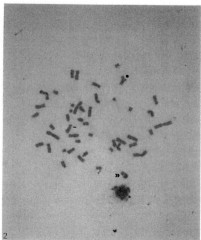

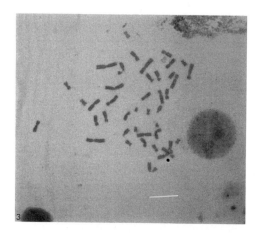

**Figure 8.1**   Chromosomal aberration test. (1) Normal karyotype; (2) Abnormal karyotype
\* – Triradial: three-armed configuration
\> \> – Ring
~ – Chromatid break
(3) Abnormal karyotype – Complex rearrangement: exchange as a result of several breaks
Original magnifications: ×1125

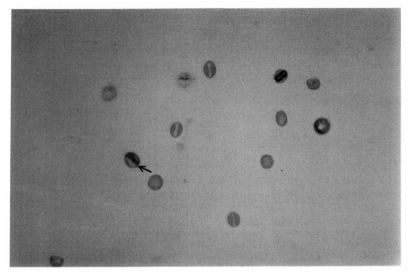

**Figure 8.2** Micronucleus test in mice – polychromatic erythrocyte with micronucleus (–>) coexisting with normal erythrocytes. Original magnification: ×450

## 8.2.4    REPAIR ASSAYS (Pedley *et al.*, 1980)

These assays demonstrate that test chemicals either cause DNA repair to occur or cause damage which can be repaired by DNA repair pathways. Thus they do not directly demonstrate mutational events, but show that a test chemical can cause the first step in the process leading to mutation.

With bacteria and yeasts this can be achieved by exposing wild-type strains, and isogenic strains deficient in DNA repair pathways, to the test chemical. If the survival of the wild-type strain is significantly greater than that of the repair-deficient strain, it can be implied that the differential killing is the result of damage to DNA. More sophisticated bacterial tests, e.g. the 'chomotest' rely on features of the so-called 'SOS' repair system. Damage to bacterial DNA by many chemicals induces activity of this repair system, which is unfortunately prone to misrepairing DNA sequences and thus leads to mutations. In the process of induction a variety of other cellular genes are also activated, and the test systems use these to provide easy methods of detecting SOS induction.

DNA repair can also be studied in mammalian cells. Cell cultures must first be pretreated to prevent normal cell division and DNA replication, e.g. with hydroxyurea. The cells are then exposed to the test substance (with and without a metabolising system) in the presence of a radiolabelled DNA precursor, tritiated thymidine. After an appropriate treatment period the cells are harvested and the extent of tritium uptake into the cellular DNA is determined. An increase in tritium uptake as a result of the test chemical treatment is taken as evidence of DNA repair synthesis; the test is referred to as 'unscheduled DNA synthesis'.

**Table 8.2** Initial classification of substances through dual genotoxicity studies

| *In vivo* micronucleus test or metaphase analysis | Ames test | Conclusion |
|---|---|---|
| + | + | Certainly a carcinogen |
| − | − | Certainly a non-carcinogen – to be confirmed |
| + | − | Certainly a carcinogen |
| − | + | Complementary tests necessary |

### 8.2.5 SIGNIFICANCE OF MUTAGENICITY TESTS FOR EVALUATING MEDICAL DEVICES

A number of mechanisms may lead to the presence of reactive chemicals in the use of medical devices:

* migration and leaching of trace constituents, including residual, monomers, plasticisers, additives etc.
* exposure during the unpolymerised phase
* degradation, leading to the production of toxic metabolites.

Since the demonstration of the relationship between carcinogenic and mutagenic effects on the Ames test (McCann *et al.*, 1976), the correlation between long-term carcinogenicity tests in animals and short-term mutagenicity tests has been established in the range of 50–70%. However, this correlation may vary according to the chemical classification.

Genotoxicity studies are aimed at being used as 'screening' tests to eliminate mutagenic substances which are potentially carcinogenic. It has been shown (Shelby and Zeigler, 1990) that all the substances of Group 1 of the IARC are detected by two tests, namely the Ames test and the rodent bone marrow cytogenic test. Thus these two tests allow a first classification and the most dangerous substances may be eliminated (Table 8.2).

They should be complemented by other tests in order to verify that the effect:

* observed on bacteria is verified on mammal cells
* is not related to organ specificity
* is really due to DNA lesion rather than to methodological bias.

Most mutagens require metabolic conversion to an active metabolite. Usually *in vitro* tests employ a microsomal preparation of induced rodent liver to which adequate cofactors have been added. Greater importance should be given to those mutagens that prove active in live animals, than to those that are only positive *in vitro*. A negative result *in vitro* is totally devoid of significance if parallel positive results are obtained *in vivo*. Some of the technical artefacts that can give rise to false positive results are changes in osmolarity and pH causing toxicity.

## 8.3  CARCINOGENICITY

### 8.3.1  GENERAL CONSIDERATIONS

Most biomaterials are able to promote tumour formation in rodents; most of them contain components – or are derived from components or degrade to yield components – which are known to be chemical carcinogens. However, very few cases of tumour have been reported with respect to the clinical use of implantable medical devices. There is therefore a major problem in the introduction of new biomaterials, as they must be tested for carcinogenicity without any acceptable and validated test procedure that is predictive of clinical performance.

Experimental evidence (Pedley *et al.*, 1980) indicates that metals and plastics can induce malignant neoplasms in laboratory animals. Tumour incidence is influenced by the species and strain of the animals used, and also the physical form and particle size in which the materials are implanted. With polymers or ceramics, larger solid implants generally give rise to a greater incidence of tumours than do particulate or powdered material (Brand *et al.*, 1967; Brand, 1994). However, some materials can also induce experimental tumours because of their chemical composition. This solid-state carcinogenesis has become known as the Oppenheimer effect, after the description in the 1950s of the phenomenon of 'polymer' or 'foreign-body carcinogenesis'. Plastics and various other solid materials have been shown to cause sarcomas in rats and mice at subcutaneous and intraperitoneal implantation sites (Oppenheimer *et al.*, 1948, 1961) (Figures 8.3–8.5).

They have been associated with the nature of the fibrotic response and fibrous capsule formation. In general, chemical carcinogenesis has been assumed to be of minor importance in comparison to this solid-state physical effect, but the increased incidence of tumours with particulate metal could be related to chemical carcinogenesis as a result of the release of metal ions from a large surface area (Oppenheimer *et al.*, 1956). Chemical carcinogenesis is a complex phenomenon related to the access of the carcinogen to appropriate intracellular structures, usually considered to be DNA (but possibly also other targets), as described in Section 8.2 and in Chapter 6 Part II.

However, the clinical evidence concerning the risks of tumour formation following implantation of materials remains very sparse. Occasionally authors have shown the possibility of a causal relationship between prosthesis and tumour, but there tends to have been a considerable underreporting of such cases. One study attempted to correlate remote tumours with devices in a statistical and epidemiological survey (Gillespie *et al.*, 1988). A significant decrease was observed in the general cancer incidence up to 10 years after implantation, in contrast to a significant increase observed in patients surviving more than 10 years. The risk ranged from 2% in the whole population to 6% in the operated group.

Any discussion about the specificity of the Oppenheimer effect should also

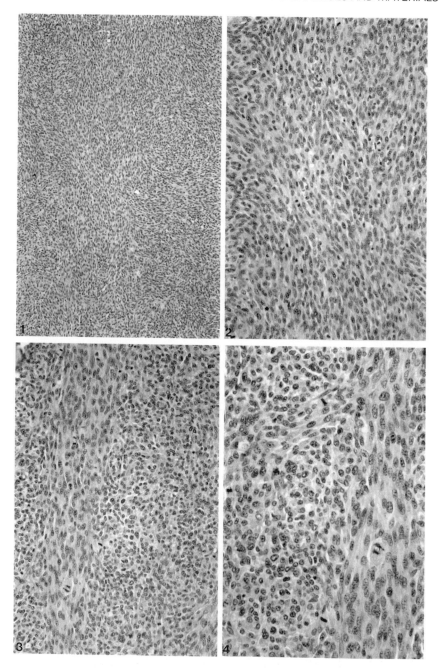

**Figure 8.3** Polyethylene-induced subcutaneous tumour in a rat after 29 weeks' implantation – fibrosarcoma. Original magnifications: 1. × 112, 2. × 281, 3. × 281, 4. × 450

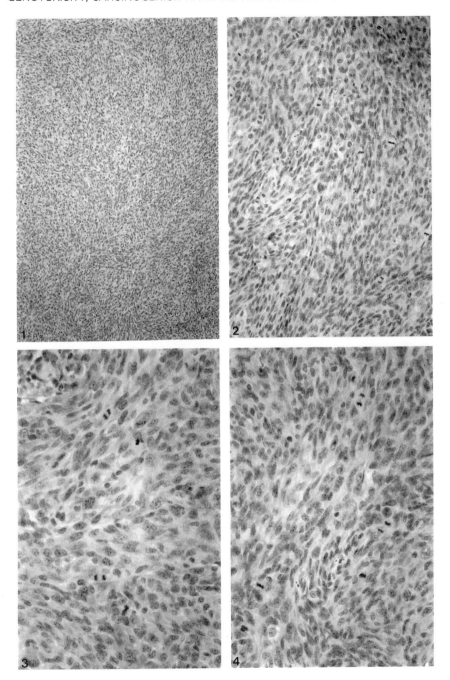

**Figure 8.4** Titanium-induced subcutaneous tumour in a rat after 50 weeks' implantation – fibrosarcoma. Original magnifications: 1. × 45, 2. × 112, 3. × 281, 4. × 281

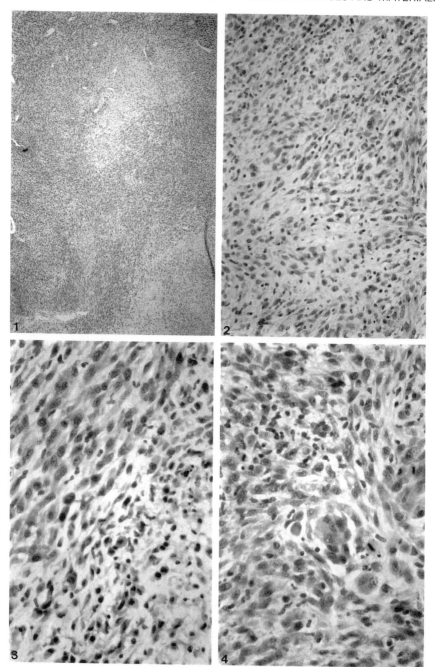

**Figure 8.5**  Polyurethane-induced subcutaneous tumour in the rat after 44 weeks' implantation. Large heterogeneous fibrocytes/ macrophages/lymphocytes populations with giant multinucleated cells, high mitotic rate – malignant fibrous histiosarcoma. Original magnifications: 1. × 45, 2. × 281, 3. × 281, 4. × 450

include the difference in incidences of tumour formation among different materials of similar shape and size, or among different kinds of chemical structures of some polymers (Nakamura, 1992). The possibility of the development of neoplasia in rodents due to mechanical irritation has also been discussed.

The requirement to evaluate the potential for new materials to evoke a neoplastic response is generally reserved for those materials which have not previously been used for human implantation for a significant period of time. Genotoxicity assays may be initiated and proposed as an alternative to an *in vivo* tumorigenicity bioassay, but they may also be considered as initial screening procedures owing to their sensitivity, the significantly reduced time needed to obtain valuable data, and the desire to reduce the use of animals for testing (ASTM, 1992). According to ISO 10993-3, situations suggesting the need for carcinogenicity testing may include the following:

- resorbable materials and devices, unless there are significant and adequate data on human use or exposure
- materials and devices where positive results have been obtained in genetic toxicity.

## 8.3.2  DESIGN CONSIDERATIONS FOR A CARCINOGENICITY EVALUATION

Criteria that should be considered in method design are as follows:

- choice of animal model
  Mice are not recommended for testing biomaterials because their small size is inappropriate for the placement of solid implants. Fischer 344 rats and other strains (Sprague–Dawley, Long Evans or Wistar) have been recommended. Both sexes should be used unless the device will ultimately be used only in males or females.
- selection of implant size and form
  The ratio of implant surface area to body volume should be in excess of the anticipated dosages observed in clinical practice. An extract should not be used as a substitute for the material to be tested. The physical form and properties of the implant should be carefully addressed owing to their impact on tumorigenesis and should be representative of the intended end-use, including debris or wear particles, if appropriate.
- a dose–response effect should be considered whenever possible
- control groups
  These should be animals which have undergone a sham operating procedure, but owing to the previously described difficulties in interpreting tumours at the implant site an additional group should include animals receiving a selected, appropriate negative reference material.
- size of the test groups
  The number of animals in each group shall be adequate for statistical analysis of the risk to be addressed and regulatory purposes. The National toxicology

programme requires 60 animals/sex/group for chemical studies, with 10 animals being sacrificed earlier than 2 years. Other recommendations or publications utilise 30–50 animals/sex/group.

- duration of the study (recommended to be 2 years)
- evaluation of the results

The test and control animals are carefully examined twice weekly, with a complete record of their clinical status and any mass appearance and development being maintained. At termination or early death, or sacrifice for humane considerations, a complete necropsy should be performed and any abnormalities or lesions should be noted and evaluated by histopathology. A minimal and a complementary list of tissues to be evaluated by histopathology also includes the implant site and the lymph nodes in the region of the implant.

It should be noted, however, that the cost, length and relative clinical relevance of carcinogenicity testing is one of the major drawbacks to the actual development of new biomaterials.

### 8.3.3  SIGNIFICANCE OF CARCINOGENICITY STUDIES

The relevance to carcinogenesis of the alteration of the immune system induced by leachables from a medical device also remains to be elucidated. Their interaction with antitumour mechanisms, e.g. NK cells and macrophages, as well as the site of the interaction, should be investigated in any established protocol(s). Different animal species or strains can respond differently to the immunomodulatory activity of chemicals. The interaction of these chemicals with the mechanisms of natural tumoricidal activity is also very heterogeneous.

Comparative evaluations have been undertaken to establish to what extent data on a particular chemical obtained in short-term mutagenicity tests are consistent with the results achieved when the same compound is investigated in long-term animal studies: 90% of a total of 175 chemicals were simultaneously mutagenic and carcinogenic, whereas the remaining 10% were so-called 'false negatives', i.e. carcinogenic but not mutagenic. Of 108 chemicals known to be non-carcinogens, 13% proved to be mutagens. However, several studies agree on one major point, namely that there are certain compounds undetected in the short-term tests which are carcinogenic in both humans and animals. None of the short-term assays so far employed have been shown to be totally satisfactory for predicting the carcinogenic potential of all chemicals tested. It is therefore recommended to use a battery of tests and at least two species for *in vivo* testing, and the interpretation of the results should account for the number of responses in a given direction.

## 8.4  REPRODUCTIVE TOXICITY TESTS

These tests should normally be considered for the following types of medical devices:

- intrauterine devices (IUDs), or any other long-term contact device likely to come into direct contact with reproductive tissues or the embryo/fetus
- energy-depositing devices
- resorbable or leachable materials and devices.

IUDs, resorbable devices or devices containing leachable moieties shall be tested in their 'ready-to-use' form. The maximum implantable dose (MID) of a material or device should be applied. Where possible, this dose should be expressed as a multiple of the worst case. Assessment of effects should be made based on absorption-kinetic data and the following modifications considered:

- dose
- route of application
- exposure time.

The material should be implanted for a period which allows for the distribution of any corrosion, leachable or degradation products, prior to insemination. The human route of exposure should be mimicked and surgical stress to the animals during pregnancy should also be avoided. Fecundity and fertility should be evaluated at levels equivalent to a reasonably large human exposure. Serial mating procedures should be continued until a sufficient number ($>25$) of sperm-positive females can be assigned to each dose group.

Animals are observed daily for clinical signs of toxicity. Mean food weights and body weights are recorded for the animals in each group every 2–3 days until day 20. At this time the animals are killed and examined for maternal liver and uterus weights, implant status, fetal weight, sex and morphological development. Pregnancy rates are compared in control and treated groups. The frequency of postimplantation loss, mean fetal body weight/litter, and prevalence of external, visceral or skeletal malformations is established. Depending on the intended human use and material characteristics, pre-/postnatal studies may be indicated. If information derived from other tests indicates potential effects on the male reproduction system, then appropriate tests for male reproductive toxicity shall be conducted.

## 8.5  CONCLUSION

These three topics form an important area where, even today, there is still room for:

- an improved understanding of the basic mechanisms leading up to, and involved in, genetic alteration or increased incidence of neoplastic formation
- improved and validated standardised short-term tests which can be relied upon to predict long-term effects and clinical performance.

Some of the most promising current research is centred on a molecular biology approach, but it is still early to report even preliminary data.

## 8.6 REFERENCES

Ames BN, McCann J and Yamasaki E (1975) Methods for detecting carcinogens and mutagens with the *Salmonella*/mammalian microsome mutagenicity test. Mutat Res 31:437.

ASTM F-1439 (1992) standard guide for performance of a lifetime bioassay for the tumorigenic potential of implant materials, 11.04. ASTM, Philadelphia, USA.

Brand GK (1994) Do implanted medical devices cause cancer? J Biomat Appl 8:325–343.

Brand GK, Buoen LC and Brand I (1967) Carcinogenesis from polymer implants: new aspects from chromosome and transplantation studies during pre-malignancy. J Natl Cancer Inst 39:663.

Forster R (1986) Mutagenicity testing and biomaterials. In: Williams DF (ed) Techniques of biocompatibility testing II. CRC Press, Boca Raton, Florida, USA.

Gillespie WF, Frampton CMA and Henderson RJ (1988) The incidence of cancer following total hip replacement. J Bone Joint Surg 70B:539–542.

ISO (1994) Biological evaluation of medical devices, Part 3. Tests for genotoxicity, carcinogenicity and reproductive toxicity. ISO, Geneva, Switzerland.

McCann J, Choi E, Yamasaki E and Ames B (1976) Detection of carcinogens and mutagens in the *Salmonella*/microsome test: assay of 300 chemicals, I. Proc Natl Acad Sci USA 72:5135 & II. Proc Natl Acad Sci USA 73:950.

Nakamura A (1992) Difference in tumour incidence and other tissue responses to polyetherurethane and polydimethylsiloxane in long-term subcutaneous implantation into rats. J Biomed Mat Res 26:631–650.

Oppenheimer BS, Oppenheimer ET and Stout AP (1948) Sarcomas induced in rats by implanting cellophane. Proc Soc Exp Biol Med 67:33.

Oppenheimer BS, Oppenheimer ET, Danishefsky I and Stout AP (1956) Carcinogenic effect of metals in rodents. Cancer Res 16:439.

Oppenheimer ET, Wilihite M, Danishefsky I and Stout AP (1961) Observations on the effects of powdered polymer in the carcinogenic process. Cancer Res 21:132.

Pedley B, Meachim G and Williams DF (1980) Tumour induction by implant materials. In: Williams DF (ed) Fundamental aspects of biocompatibility II. CRC Press, Boca Raton, Florida, USA.

Shelby MD and Zeigler MD (1990) Activity of human carcinogens in the *Salmonella* and rodent bone marrow cytogenetic tests. Mutat Res 234:257–262.

# 9
# Explant Retrieval and Analysis

JAGDISH BUTANY
Department of Pathology, The Toronto Hospital and University of Toronto,
Toronto, Canada

## 9.1  INTRODUCTION

Bioprosthetic devices have a long history of generally safe and satisfactory use. Much of the current knowledge of biological events, occurring as part of the host tissue and biomaterial response to implanted prosthetic devices, is based on painstaking studies by numerous individuals working with a combination of experimental data and clinical retrieval studies (surgical explants and removal at autopsy).

In spite of significant improvements in biomaterials technology, and the development and improved durability of biomaterials (and bioprosthetic devices made from them), they are not yet perfect. Prostheses-related complications continue to occur and significantly affect patient prognosis following the implant of such devices. Detailed examination and analysis of explanted prosthetic devices is therefore critical.

Properly performed and systematic evaluations of explanted prosthetic devices lead to increasing knowledge – e.g. rates, morphologic features and mechanisms – of prosthesis-related complications, and so contribute to improved patient care. Furthermore, these analyses elucidate the structural basis of favourable performance and help predict the effects of future developments/modifications on device safety and efficacy. Any individual interested in the analysis of explanted biomaterials should use a systematic approach similar to that outlined in Figure 9.1.

## 9.2  OBJECTIVES

Morphological examination of bioprostheses, obtained either at autopsy or at surgical explantation, provides very valuable information. For any individual patient, determination of the cause of failure of a bioprosthesis, or elucidation of the untoward reactions to a biomaterial, can help in the future management of the

*Biocompatibility Assessment of Medical Devices and Materials.*
Edited by Julian Braybrook. © 1997 John Wiley & Sons Ltd.

**DETAILED ANALYSES OF BIOPROSTHESIS**

Name:                 Hospital #:
Age:   Yr:   Sex: M/F     Pathology #:
Location of Prosthesis:
Reason for Implantation:
Date of Implantation:
Reason for Explantation:
Date of Explantation:        Duration of Implant:
Type of Prosthesis:
Manufacturer:           Model:
Note:   1. Specimen should be fixed in appropriate medium.
        2. Specimen must be handled with latex gloves at all times.

**GROSS EXAMINATION:**
Note:    Site from which Explanted:
           Type of Bioprosthesis:
           Serial # (if available):
           Composition of Bioprosthesis:
           Presence of any Biological Tissues:
           Measure and Record appropriate Dimensions:
Note:   1. Appearance:
        2. Any Changes as compared to Pre-Implant Device:
        3. Consistency of Biological Tissues:
           a) Any hardening (? Mineralisation).
           b) Any tears. Note location.
           c) Prolapse of tissues.
           d) Any vegetations/thrombus.
           e) Pannus. Note thickness and extension on the sewing ring and cusps.

**RADIOLOGICAL EXAMINATION (2 PLANES, AT LEAST) IN A FAXITRON:**
Note:   1. Manufacturer, Device, Model # etc:
        2. Presence of Materials Damage:
           a) #.
           b) Loss of parts of device.
           c) Deposition of minerals.
           d) Check integrity of device.

**PROSTHETIC HEART VALVES:**
Gross: Type of Prosthesis:

| 1. Bioprosthesis: | 2. Mechanical: |
|---|---|
| Porcine: Carpentier-Edwards. | Starr-Edwards. |
| Hancock I. | Bjork-Shiley. |
| Hancock II. | St. Jude Medical Bileaflet. |
| Hancock MO. | Medtronic-Hall. |
| Hancock Mosaic. | Othe |
| Hancock Intact. | |
| Pericardial C.E. (ISLP and Hancock – Discontinued). | |

**X-RAY:** Mineralisation.   Grade: 0,1+,2+,3+,4+
                      Location:
Measure Size of Effective Orifice:
Measure Size of Each of 3 Cusps:
Note:   a) Cusp tears.
        b) Cusp prolapse.
        c) Cusp redundancy.
        d) Pannus. Location.

**PHOTOGRAPHY:**    1. Photograph both surfaces of device.
                        2. Photograph after removal of attached tissue.
                        3. Photograph close up of special tissue.

**MICROSCOPY:**           Take sections as required.
(H&E, Gram, Von Kossa, Other)   Note orientation and location of cut tissue.
                                 Analyse section.

**DIAGNOSIS:**

**COMMENTS:** Summarise findings and correlate with clinical features.

**Figure 9.1** Systematic approach recommended for detailed analysis of explanted biomaterials

patient and diagnosis of infections (e.g. infective endocarditis in prosthetic heart valves). This allows the use of appropriate medications, especially antibiotics. Often, the surgeon requests intraoperative pathological consultation when working on a bioprosthesis. This may help decide the type of replacement device to be used (a bioprosthesis vs a mechanical heart valve prosthesis, for example, or vice versa).

In spite of the fact that numerous *in vitro* tests for durability and biocompatibility, as well as animal investigations, are undertaken before clinical use of prosthetic devices, pathological analyses of explanted prosthetic devices (especially cohorts of explanted devices) help in the determination of their safety and efficacy. Often these investigations will document changes well beyond those determined by previous tests. This contributes to improved clinical recognition of complications and helps guide future development of prosthetic devices. In addition to explanted human devices, pathologists are often called upon to evaluate devices implanted in animal models (e.g. dogs, sheep or pigs), so that the manufacturer can predict the effects of potentially useful modifications to materials and designs.

Pathologists play a significant regulatory role in recognising clinical prosthesis-associated complications as specified by the US Medical Devices Act 1990 (PL101-629). This legislation has specific user reporting requirements which require that healthcare personnel in hospitals report all device-related deaths, significant illness and injury, to the US FDA or the manufacturer, or both (depending on the nature of the incident). Similar requirements are in place in Canada and several other countries. Where no such requirements exist as yet, legislation is likely to occur in the future. Thus a scientist or pathologist who makes such initial discovery of significant malfunction or death of an individual, relatable to a bioprosthetic device, must initiate the reporting process.

The objectives of analysis of explanted bioprosthetic devices can therefore be summarised as:

- development of better patient selection criteria for improved matching of patient and prosthesis
- recognition and documentation of device-related complications
- progressive improvement in the development of prostheses and the elimination of specific complications
- documentation of early and late changes in bioprostheses
- documentation and a better understanding of the tissue–biomaterial interactions
- assessment of the efficacy and benefit of improvements/changes in prosthesis design
- compliance with the mandatory device reporting regulation requirements (of the FDA, 1984).

## 9.3 SPECIMEN HANDLING

All explanted biomaterials should be examined in detail by a pathologist, preferably one with an interest in prosthetic devices and biomaterials. In the absence of such an individual the manufacturer will usually be willing to examine the explanted device, at his expense, and issue a report on it. Each specimen should be examined with the appropriate clinical information available. This should include the following:

- reasons for the implant
- the duration of the implant
- reasons for explantation
- type of replacement device implanted at the second surgery.

These prosthetic devices may be purely synthetic, i.e. composed only of:

- man-made materials, such as polymers or different types of metals and alloys
- a combination of biologic materials mounted on artificial stents
- purely biological materials.

When handling these, one must follow a systematic approach. In all cases, if there is any suspicion of infection the first step (prior to any further handling) should be to take a swab from the appropriate area and send it for microbiological culture. In the case of biological tissues, if vegetations are seen on the tissue, pieces of the vegetation and the underlying tissue should be sent for microbiological examination. Microbiological examination should include cultures for aerobic and non-aerobic organisms. Devices such as vascular implants made of polytetrafluoroethylenes (PTFE and ePTFE) may require specific handling, and for this the materials must immediately be placed in cold buffered glutaraldehyde (2.5%), especially if electron microscopy is to be performed. All specimens must be treated as potentially infected and therefore handled with appropriate care (universal precautions); latex gloves must be worn. The materials must be placed in the appropriate fixative for an adequate period of time (generally 24 hours) before examination.

There are many protocols available for examination of different devices. Further protocols are being developed by many groups interested in prosthetic devices. These include the US FDA, ISO, and the Association for Advancement of Medical Instrumentation (AAMI). In addition to these, many laboratories have their own protocols (Figure 9.1). The great advantage of using a protocol is the minimisation of the likelihood of missing any step in the analytical process.

A permanent record of changes observed in the device must be kept: this includes photographing all prosthetic devices on all surfaces. If possible (especially in biomaterials without synthetic components), when examining hollow devices, e.g. vascular grafts, the cut surfaces of the specimens should also be photographed. The specimen should then be examined in detail and gross features recorded, using the available protocol.

## 9.4 TECHNIQUES FOR THE EXAMINATION OF EXPLANTED BIOMATERIALS

### 9.4.1 INTRODUCTION

There are many different techniques available for the examination of explanted devices, but not all of them are required in every instance. For obvious reasons, more of these are used in the analysis of investigative devices than for those in regular, more or less routine, usage. Perhaps the most common, cheap and useful investigation is gross examination. Light microscopy can provide a wealth of crucial information about the device and the host response to it. With adequate information, and when performed by a knowledgeable person, this examination can be invaluable. The protocol for examination must include information regarding the patient's age, sex and the procedure performed. The patient's age at the time of implant is essential, as some changes occur very rapidly at certain patient ages. Patient's condition prior to implant, reason for implantation, implant site, reason for explantation and the implant duration are other essential pieces of information. The name of the manufacturer and the lot and serial numbers of the implant can provide significant preimplantation information about the device; if the device failed, whether similar failures have occurred in other similar devices would assist the documentation process. The name of the physician and his address and telephone number should also be available.

### 9.4.2 GROSS EXAMINATION

Before starting the evaluation of a device it is desirable to have a good idea of the appearance of the preimplanted device. The gross examination is a detailed visual appraisal of the device. It is the most critical stage of the analysis, because once the device is cut its features cannot be recreated. Photography will provide some data, but not all the information of a competent and complete gross examination: no photograph will convey the consistency, flexibility and pliability of a biological tissue.

The gross evaluation should include the measurements of different dimensions and the morphologic appearance of the explanted device. Some information regarding the preimplant features of the device are obviously extremely helpful in identifying postimplant changes, e.g. the ball in a Starr–Edwards prosthesis changes colour from white to golden yellow after years of use.

Specific note must be made of:

- the presence of sutures or other anchoring material
- the colour of the device
- the results of digital or visual evaluation of the mechanical integrity of the device
- the results of digital evaluation of the nature of the tissue (the pliability of biological tissues, e.g. bioprosthetic heart valves)

- the range and ease of movement of the different moving parts of a device (e.g. prosthetic heart valves)
- any tissue capsule around the prosthetic device (e.g. pacemakers and pacemaker leads)
- whether there are any vegetations adherent to any part of the device (a significant feature for prosthetic heart valves)
- any host tissue growth into, or on to, the device (e.g. vascular grafts and prosthetic heart valves)
- the presence of external rings (e.g. orthopaedic devices)
- evidence of any infection, i.e. purulent material adherent to the device (e.g. an annular abscess around prosthetic valves)
- any abnormal bulges in the contour of the device (e.g. pseudoaneurysms or aneurysms forming around a vascular graft or at its junction with the native vessel)
- the examination of the device using a stereodissection microscope (often helpful for noting changes in small devices and surface changes in larger ones).

### 9.4.3 RADIOGRAPHY

Most devices containing metal components are examined radiologically. The majority of these devices are fairly small and are best examined in a Faxitron, i.e. a desktop X-ray machine that is small, safe and convenient to use. It uses the same type of film as that used in hospital radiology departments and provides excellent specimen radiographs. It assists with documentation of the integrity of the metallic component of the device, noting any abnormalities such as evidence of fracture and/or mineralisation in biological tissues or tissues around the device. In orthopaedic devices, if the bone is removed with the implant the radiograph helps record changes in the bone itself. X-ray examination of explanted bioprosthetic heart valves and orthopaedic devices is essential: not only does it help decide on device integrity and the presence of mineralisation, if any, it also often allows determination of the type of prosthesis, i.e. its identification and specific brand (Figure 9.2).

### 9.4.4 LIGHT MICROSCOPY

Obviously, light microscopy is not feasible with many bioprostheses, e.g. those composed of metals or polymers alone, and is therefore utilised only for the host tissue adherent to the device or the biological component of the prosthetic device. Tissues to be processed for light microscopy are fixed in 10% buffered formalin and, typically after 24 hours, embedded in paraffin (or plastic) prior to cutting into sections of 3–5 $\mu$m thickness. The advantage of paraffin embedding is that it is cheap, all laboratories are equipped to handle it, and many more special stains (including immunohistochemical stains) can be used on these sections. The advantage of plastic (e.g. glycol methylmethacrylate, GMMA)-embedded sections is that the tissues can be examined without having to be decalcified. Furthermore,

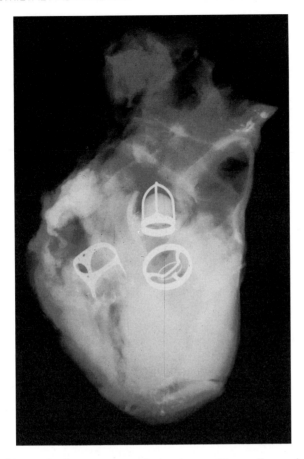

**Figure 9.2** X-ray of a heart removed at autopsy. The radiograph shows three different kinds of prosthetic heart valves in three different sites. The tricuspid valve shows a standard model Ionescu–Shiley valve. The mitral site shows a Bjork–Shiley tilting disc, monostrut valve (now the Sorin Biomedical Valve). In the aortic site is a Starr–Edwards prosthesis. These prostheses were implanted several years ago and the patient died of unrelated causes. The apical end of the heart shows small foci of mineralisation, related to previous surgical procedures. The Ionescu–Shiley prosthesis in the tricuspid position is a biological prosthesis (bovine pericardium mounted on a synthetic frame and held in place with Dacron fabric). The Starr–Edwards and the Bjork–Shiley monostrut prostheses are mechanical valves, being composed entirely of synthetic materials

some synthetic materials (e.g. fabrics) are easier to cut and their relationships to adjacent tissues is better preserved.

The cut sections are mounted on glass slides and stained, typically with haematoxylin and eosin, to allow differentiation of the cell cytoplasm and nucleus, the connective tissues, nerves, vessels etc. For the definitive differentiation of tissue components, e.g. connective tissues from epithelial tissues and elastic tissues in vascular materials, additional histological stains can be utilised. The elastic trichrome stain (a combination of Verhoeff van Gieson and Masson trichrome) and the Movat Pentachrome stain are especially useful for vascular grafts and graft–native vessel junctions. If there is any suspicion of infection, or if the patient was known clinically to have had graft or prosthesis infection, the soft tissues removed at the time of the surgical procedure must be stained for microorganisms in addition to being submitted for microbiological examination. The common stains used are Gram's stain for bacteria, and the PAS and GMS stains for fungi. Today, new immunohistochemical stains and *in situ* hybridisation techniques are available for detecting small numbers of many microorganisms, e.g. cytomegalovirus or other viruses, in addition to light microscopy.

Tissues prepared for light microscopy may be examined by transmitted light (the usual form of light microscopy) or incident light. The latter way is used for thick sections, where light cannot pass through the specimen and light is instead shone directly on the surface being examined. In addition, polarised light should be used when examining prosthetic materials, as foreign materials and materials trapped in macrophages and other cells are much more easily identified, being birefringent.

## 9.4.5  IMMUNOHISTOCHEMISTRY

Further detailed characterisation of tissue cells often requires immunohistochemical studies (Bienz and Egger, 1995; Eichmeller *et al.*, 1996; Jensen *et al.*, 1996; Sheild *et al.*, 1996). These confirm the nature of otherwise non-typical or poorly differentiated tissues, e.g. those reacting to foreign devices. Depending on the type of bioprosthesis and biomaterial(s), the host reaction varies. In devices implanted in the cardiovascular system, it is often essential to decide whether the surface of the biomaterials was endothelialised or not. For this, immunohistochemical stains, e.g. Factor VIII or *Ulex Europaeus*, are frequently helpful. In explants it is often necessary to decide the type of cell responding to the biomaterials. In cardiovascular implants, these are often less differentiated vascular smooth muscle cells. Here smooth muscle actin and other similar immunohistochemical stains are helpful, although these cells differentiate further to produce collagen, and at that time stains for fibroblasts may be required as the smooth muscle stains may be negative. In the early postimplantation period, i.e. within a few weeks (up to 10), a larger number of immunohistochemical stains are necessary to type these cells, because at this time the responding cells may be macrophages, smooth muscle-derived cells, endothelial cells or other inflammatory cells. In addition, it is at times necessary to decide whether the cells are replicating, and at this stage the PCNA stain is often helpful.

## 9.4.6  MORPHOMETRIC ANALYSIS

Morphometric analysis using simple attachments to a light microscope or, for greater accuracy, a computerised image analysis system attached to the microscope, allows the quantification of changes in explanted devices. With this approach, the analyst can gauge the exact degree of host tissue response to a device, e.g. measurement of changes in the (inner) flow surface in a vascular graft provides a good indication of the functional status of the graft while *in situ*; the exact location of the changes may help decide the need for changes in configuration, design and anastomoses of the device. The same process can be used to measure the thickness of the prosthetic device and determine whether any part of it has been lost or destroyed. The thickness of the inflammatory and tissue responses on the outer surface can be gauged by the same process.

### 9.4.7 'NEW RESEARCH' TECHNOLOGIES

Many newer tests and characterisation methodologies are currently in use. These include flow cytometry, DNA analysis and *in situ* hybridisation. Most of these are still primarily used in basic sciences and are not easily adaptable or available for the everyday clinical situation; one of the major limiting factors is the associated cost. In the case of tissue implants, e.g. homograft heart valves (fresh or frozen), such tests can help determine whether the cells in the tissue are from the host or the donor, and whether the implanted tissue is viable or 'dead'.

Immunohistochemical studies help identify specific cells and determine the activity of the cell in accordance with enzyme production and activation. These can be reliably and reproducibly employed in the experimental as well as the clinical setting.

### 9.4.8 ELECTRON MICROSCOPY

Where the tissues are to be examined by electron microscopy, specimens are immersed in cold buffered 2.5% glutaraldehyde or universal fixative for either transmission (TEM) or scanning (SEM) electron microscopy. SEM allows surface (and surface changes) characterisation of tissues. In this procedure, the fixed tissue's surface is critical-point dried and coated with either gold or carbon. The surface is then examined and any change documented. A basic understanding of cardiac ultrastructure, structure and pathology is critical prior to undertaking these studies.

X-ray diffraction microanalysis helps determine the types of particles present in the tissue being examined, the different components easily being identified. X-ray defraction (XRD) studies may be helpful in selected materials (Valdre *et al.*, 1995). However, these studies do not identify the specific elements, their location, or the cellular effects in the human patient. Atomic force microscopy and immunoelectron microscopy are other methods for the study of fine biological structures (Moore, 1995; Moreira *et al.*, 1996). Analytical electron microscopy can identify individual materials and locate these within the various organelles of the cell (electron energy loss spectroscopy) (Ferrans and Butany, 1983). However, both techniques are expensive and difficult and are therefore not used on a routine basis.

## 9.4.9   WHOLE SPECIMEN ANALYSIS

It is increasingly important to be able to examine the intact interface between biomaterials and their surrounding tissues. This applies to virtually all prosthetic devices, but is significant in the case of orthopaedic and cardiovascular devices, especially those where there is a biological component in the device itself. It is also important in some dental and mammary implants. Relatively few centres have the ability to examine the whole specimen, i.e. without having to remove the synthetic/metal components. In general, this process involves the embedding of the whole specimen, e.g. the head of the femur (but not the whole of the attached shaft of the prosthesis), in plastic (e.g. GMMA or PMNA), which is then allowed to harden or cure for 4–6 weeks. The embedded specimen is cut to the appropriate thickness using a high-precision diamond bandsaw. The surface of the section (0.5–1.0 cm in thickness) is mounted on a thick glass slide, ground, polished and stained with haematoxylin and eosin, or one of a few other stains. The specimen is examined with incident light and a complete and detailed analysis performed (Butany *et al.*, 1990). This process helps determine any surface changes in the prosthetic material and any changes in the adjoining tissues. The surface changes must be photographically recorded, as examination of the deeper parts of the device requires further grinding of the surface and loss of the intervening material. There are a few automated systems available for this type of processing: one such is manufactured by Logitech (Struers) and consists of a precision lapping system with an aluminum slurry. A precision press is used to make the samples adhere to the slide. The sample is up to 10–15 mm thick and embedded in plastic.

## 9.5   CHANGES ASSOCIATED WITH PROSTHETIC DEVICES

### 9.5.1   TISSUE RESPONSES

Prosthetic devices are classified as being made of bioprosthetic materials. However, as has already been shown in earlier chapters, the body treats all such materials in the same way, i.e. as 'foreign'. However, the severity of the reaction varies with the bioreactivity or antigenicity of the material.

Frequently, the tissue reaction is variable and very much different from that observed in the animal used in the preclinical study. It can also vary from patient to patient, in degree if not in type, and between different areas of the interface of the implant in the same host. Resulting surface changes in the prostheses can be well characterised by a range of techniques, and especially electron spectroscopy (ESCA) (Ratner, 1983).

The major purpose of the body's defence mechanism is to attempt to remove the material by phagocytosis and enzymatic digestion, or to isolate it by the formation of a fibrous capsule. In the case of small or absorbable materials the resulting reaction soon results in their disposal. In non-absorbable materials placed as permanent implants, the implant itself remains in the body and the body aims to sequester it with varying degrees of fibrous tissue reaction and the formation of a capsule or envelope; for example, with pacemaker power packs implanted subcutaneously, or deeper, in the left subclavicular region, within a few weeks a thin but strong fibrous tissue capsule is formed around the entire device.

These changes in the host tissue include an invariable response or trauma to tissues, blood vessels and capillaries (and therefore a varying degree of haemorrhage) as a result of the surgical procedure (implantation) itself. The tissue damage and acute inflammation consequent to the surgical procedure are mediated by numerous factors, including cytokines (interleukin-1 (IL-1), tumour necrosis factor (TNF) and $\gamma$-interferon), leucocytes and macrophages (Brett and Kukatsu, 1995; Greenhalgh, 1996). The presence of macrophages is essential for the initiation and maintenance of fibroblast activity. In the initial hours following the operative procedure tissue haemorrhage and fluid accumulation occurs. This is followed by an acute inflammatory process, with hyperaemia, tissue swelling (due to oedema) and infiltration by polymorphonuclear leucocytes (Cotran, 1993; Brett and Kukatsu, 1995). This process will obviously be seen at all levels in the incised wound, and peaks within 24 hours. This inflammatory infiltrate gradually diminishes as the polymorphonuclear leucocytes disintegrate over the next 2–4 days. By 1–2 days, epithelial cells, endothelial cells and fibroblast activation are manifest in the tissue surrounding the implant, and migration and granulation tissue formation soon occur. In orthopaedic devices these fibroblasts differentiate towards chondrocytes or osteocytes by the end of the first postoperative week. At most sites, acid mucopolysaccharide-rich connective tissue will begin to appear by 1 week and mature connective (collagen) tissue is laid down by 4–6 weeks (Lingenmayer, 1992). In orthopaedic devices, the surrounding bone shows the formation of bony trabeculae and fibrocartilage within 2 weeks. After this, the tissues gradually mature and the hyperaemia diminishes. At times, the tissue around the 'foreign body' becomes calcified and/or ossified (Figures 9.3 and 9.4).

A recognisable grey-white scar or fibrous tissue capsule can then be observed surrounding the device and extending for a short distance into the adjacent normal tissues (Cotran *et al.*, 1994). Barring the occurrence of infection, all these wounds heal by first intention.

Commonly used biologically acceptable prostheses produce responses which are more or less characteristic of the materials employed to manufacture them. However, there are certain additional factors which must be borne in mind, e.g. the chemical and physical processes used in the manufacturing processes. These may involve the use of additional reagents which may not be constituents of the implanted materials. One must therefore be able to differentiate the reaction to the pure biomaterial from that due to incidental contaminants from the manufacturing process. These are often unrecognised, and usually unacknowledged, contaminants of variable quantity (Fornasier and Cameron, 1994), their presence going undetected or unstated by the manufacturer. Mechanical stresses such as those induced by physical movement of the device (resulting from movement of the host) or movement of fluids in or around the device, induce further changes

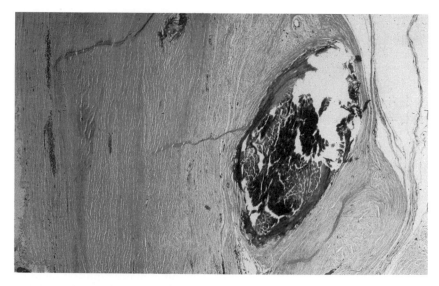

**Figure 9.3**   A Dacron ring implanted for a long period. The homogeneous tissue around it is collagen. A ring of calcification is observable around the material

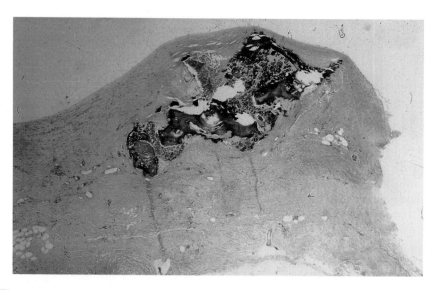

**Figure 9.4**   A synthetic suture implanted for a long period. The homogeneous tissue around it is collagen. An irregularly shaped area of ossification or bone formation is observable around the synthetic material

which may be functionally significant or insignificant, i.e. it can add an extra dimension to the resulting tissue response (often tissue adaptation and, at times, prosthesis adaptation). In the case of prosthetic orthopaedic devices, the individual's effort to avoid stress may lead to disuse of a particular part of the bone surrounding the implant (not under load), and ultimately lead to a weakened device. In the case of a cardiac pacemaker (atrial) lead, it must be able to withstand the repeated flexing and bending induced by cardiac activity. The significance of knowledge about the device, its structure and composition cannot be overstated.

Often, therefore, there is a difference between the host response to the implant as a whole (Figure 9.5) and that resulting from small fragments released from the whole owing to implant deterioration or abrasive damage (Fornasier and Cameron, 1994) (Figure 9.6). Such fragments, which are small enough to be phagocytosed by the host's histiocytes, incite a significant response by virtue of size as well as/if not the material comprising it, in addition to, or independent of, the initial implant response. This is, at times, seen in periprosthetic tissues and regional lymph nodes, e.g. where a mammary prosthesis has been 'bleeding' (Ashley *et al.*, 1967; McGrath and Burkhhardt, 1984; Cocke and Sampson, 1987).

## 9.5.2 INFECTION

Perhaps the most dreaded changes associated with prosthetic devices is the development of infection, as it usually entails their removal. Infection can occur at any time but is much more common in the early postoperative period. The rate of infection has remained fairly constant through the last 45 or so years. However, the mortality and morbidity associated with infection have diminished, largely owing to the advent of newer and stronger antibiotics, newer diagnostic techniques, greater quality control of prosthetic devices and better surgical techniques. Once infected a prosthetic device must be removed, as it is extremely difficult to eradicate the infection completely.

In orthopaedic devices fibrocartilaginous metaplasia of the fibrous tissues occurs as they mature, and is completed in 4–6 months in adults. However, bone remodelling in the tissues immediately adjacent to the implant continues for the lifetime of the implant. Osteoblastic as well as osteoclastic activity continues, with the deposition of appositional osteoid in amounts greater than normal turnover in background bone. This most probably represents an ongoing adaptation.

At later stages, a more chronic response characterised by mononuclear cells may develop. Both acute and chronic inflammation are related to exogenous or endogenous substances, with the strongest mediator being bacterial products (Snyderman and Uhuig, 1992). This is related to breakdown products of the implant materials. The mononuclear cells attempt to phagocytose the foreign materials (Wright, 1992). The body's basic defence mechanism involves the use of leucocytes and mononuclear cells (tissue and circulating histiocytes). Most

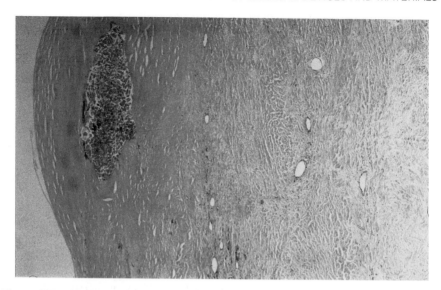

**Figure 9.5** A histologic section (haematoxylin and eosin stain) taken from close to a Dacron graft. Surrounding it is a circumferential deposit of collagen with very occasional, slim nuclei of fibroblasts visible. There has been virtually no significant inflammatory reaction to this foreign material, which is the norm rather than the exception

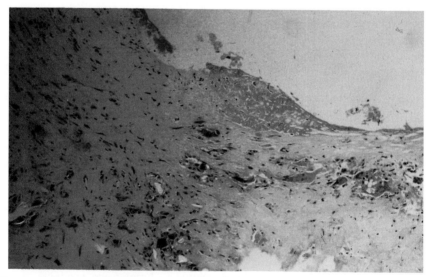

**Figure 9.6** A histologic section (haematoxlyin and eosin stain) showing a polyfilament synthetic suture. Tiny fragments or single threads of the material have broken off and incited a significant inflammatory response. The cells observed are mononuclear cells (lymphocytes and macrophages). The tiny fragments of synthetic material are surrounded by multinucleate giant cells, which are aggregates of macrophages

microorganisms or materials need to be coated by natural factors – opsonins – which bind to specific leucocyte receptors. These mononuclear cells and macrophages are a defence against infecting microorganisms as well as other foreign materials and toxic substances (Thomas and Lipsky, 1993). Histiocytes, once activated by haemostatic factors and biomaterials, attempt to destroy the foreign materials by phagocytosis and conversion of phagosomes into lysosomes. This accumulation of extracellular material (or biomaterial) within the histiocytes makes them larger and gives them a vacuolated or 'foamy' appearance. In some cases these macrophages join to form large multinucleated cells or foreign-body giant cells. When this ingested material cannot be digested, e.g. the breakdown products of synthetic implants, the cell may ultimately egest the phagosome containing this foreign material and, at the same time, release the enzymes contained in it (called the lysosomes). This foreign material, now released into the interstitium, can once again be phagocytosed by other histiocytes. The enzymes released during this process can digest the surrounding tissues and initiate further inflammatory response, as well as weakening the connective tissue or matrix that forms the supporting structure in the implant zone or the peri-implant zone. In addition to weakening the matrix, and possibly the implant itself, this allows the migration of cells attracted by the chemotactic effects of the enzymes released by the macrophages. By mechanisms not clearly understood, this also leads to activation of osteoclasts in the surrounding bone and associated increased bone reabsorption. Similar changes can be induced by bacterial infection. Somewhat similar changes are observable when silicone breast implants are either punctured or 'bleed': the foreign material incites a similar histiocytic response – engulfment of the silicone by the host macrophages – and, in time, some of these macrophages may be found in the regional (axillary) lymph nodes.

Other locally occurring changes associated with the device may be related to:

- infection: as it subsides it can result in a much greater degree of fibrosis around the implant and may lead to malfunction
- intimal reaction and fibrosis: a significant amount of intimal or endocardial fibrosis, which often extends on to the prosthetic materials (the luminal surface of the vascular graft, the sewing ring of the prosthetic heart valve or the tip of a pacemaker lead), can be incited at the junction of the graft material with the native vessel. If significant, this can lead to prosthesis dysfunction and necessitate implant removal.

Other local changes, specific to prosthetic heart valves and vascular grafts, include thrombosis, bleeding and embolic complications.

### 9.5.2.1 Thrombosis

Immediately after exposure of a prosthetic heart valve to flowing blood, a small amount of thrombus is deposited on the cloth-covered sewing ring. This is both desirable and probably beneficial. In time, host tissue grows across and through the cloth, covering it with fibrous tissue and a surface layer of endothelial cells (giving rise to a neointima). Occasional mononuclear cells and multinucleated giant cells may be seen, probably as a response to the synthetic cloth. This, theoretically at least, could lead to a reduction in thrombosis and thromboembolic phenomenon.

However, growth of thrombus on any part of the cardiovascular prosthesis could be dangerous as parts of it could disintegrate (and give rise to thromboemboli), provide a nidus for infection (any thrombus found attached to a prosthetic device should be considered infected until proven otherwise), become organised and lead to a nodular mass, and/or obstruct movement of the prosthesis (especially its occluder). Thrombi usually form at sites of relative stasis or at interfaces of different components of the device, especially where cloth and metal meet (Davies and Tripathi, 1993). Thrombosis is a major problem with mechanical heart valve prostheses, and to minimise this patients are maintained on lifelong anticoagulation. In spite of this, present-day prostheses are associated with thrombosis rates of 0.1–5.7% per patient per year (Edmonds, 1982; Metzdorff *et al.*, 1984). This increases if the patient has atrial fibrillation or fails to maintain the anticoagulant therapy. A thrombus can form at any time after the insertion of the prosthesis.

Present-day prostheses have undergone significant manufacturing changes in an effort to eliminate foci of stasis and exposed metal surfaces, either by covering them with cloth or by coating the surfaces with pyrolytic carbon, a hard thromboresistant material. With these changes, the incidence of mechanical heart valve-associated thrombus has diminished but not disappeared (Hammermeister *et al.*, 1993); it still remains essential for patients to receive anticoagulant therapy.

### 9.5.2.2  Haemorrhage

Haemorrhage can occur at the time of implantation or soon afterwards. This may be related to inadequate haemostasis, suture loosening, damage or depletion or activation of blood components during perfusion, or inadequate neutralisation of anticoagulants. This last reason is diffuse and not confined to the operative site alone, whereas inadequate haemostasis produces haemorrhage confined to the operative site. Later haemorrhage is often related to inadequately monitored anticoagulation or infection.

### 9.5.2.3  Infections

Infections, although slowly decreasing in incidence, are still common with prosthetic devices. In the early postoperative stages the common microorganisms are the skin flora and staphylococci, including *Staph. epidermidis* (Schoen, 1995). In the later stages, although virtually any microorganism may be associated with the infection, the staphylococci and streptococci still account for over 50% of cases. Once developed, the only appropriate therapy is the removal of the prosthetic device.

## 9.6 GENERAL/SYSTEMIC COMPLICATIONS ASSOCIATED WITH BIOPROSTHETIC DEVICES

Implanted and injected non-biodegradable material can be stored in the body's reticuloendothelial system for many years. In the case of injectable material, the materials are more easily followed and identified in places such as lymph nodes, spleen, liver, lungs and bone marrow. A case in point is the information obtained from drug addicts who inject talc along with the chemical agent (talc having been used to dilute the chemical agent): the foreign material or talc goes directly to the lung, where it produces a significant reaction with foreign-body granulomata. Starch is the classic foreign material used and is identified by examination of the tissue under polarized light.

Most larger implantable devices, such as orthopaedic devices, prosthetic heart valves, mammary implants or tissue expanders, are easily detected. Breakdown of the implant in any way, and the release of finer extracellular particles, can lead to a chronic inflammatory response and enlargement of the regional lymph nodes. In most of these cases the regional lymph nodes are seldom, if ever, examined, even when the device is being explanted. These extracellular particles become coated with tissue proteins and are now much more easily identified by phagocytic cells. Once ingested by the macrophage, a phagosome forms around this foreign body. It is only when there is suspicion of a chronic infection or lymphoma that the examination of the lymph nodes becomes important.

Case reports are available regarding unpolymerised polymethylmethacrylate having entered veins and travelled into the pelvis during hip arthroplasty. Similarly, there are reports of silicone from mammary implants being found in regional lymph nodes and occasionally even further beyond (Andrews, 1996). Carbon fibres, used for hardening some implants, are probably the easiest to detect on routine examination, and are easily seen as round carbon cylinders in regional (inguinal) lymph nodes. Histologically these are often associated with a histiocytic or giant-cell response. Polyethylene particles ($> 1 \mu$m diameter) can be seen under polarised light and on stained sections that have been removed from paraffin. A recently described method using fat stains for the enhancement of such particles appears to be especially useful. In the case of prosthetic heart valves, especially older mechanical models, turbulent blood flow and the closure of the orifice by the occluder (ball or disc) led to the breakdown of red blood cells, the accumulation of haemosiderin pigment, primarily in the kidneys and to a lesser extent in the spleen and liver, and occasionally haemolytic anaemia (Falk *et al.*, 1979; Skoularigis *et al.*, 1993). This is far less common with the current generation of prosthetic heart valves, both mechanical and tissue. Systemic complications have been reported in some patients who have had breast reconstruction with silicone gel implants. In these instances, the silicone is believed to have 'bled' into the adjacent tissues and a histiocytic response (as already described) occurred; the body's reaction is believed to have incited local infection, discharging sinuses, rheumatoid disease, low-grade fever etc., although there are conflicting opinions about the role of the silicone in this (Bush, 1994). Nonetheless, a significant body of litigation has followed and, unfortunately, has led to some manufacturers withdrawing very valuable biomaterials from the market.

It is fortunate that the majority of contemporary prosthetic devices function well and do not usually cause any significant host reaction; a mild local response may be observable.

## 9.7   SPECIFIC MORPHOLOGIC FEATURES OF EXPLANTED DEVICES

### 9.7.1   INTRODUCTION

Some reactions to implanted bioprosthetic devices are common and have been listed in previous sections. Many devices, however, have specific features which result in specific morphologic reactions following implantation. Some of these occur generically with prosthetic devices and are similar to those listed above, whereas others develop when a particular type of the device is implanted. In addition, there are specific features which develop in the individual patient using a particular device. This section will review some of these more specific findings.

### 9.7.2   CARDIOVASCULAR DEVICES

An increasing array of cardiovascular bioprosthetic devices is implanted today. These range from the small prosthetic vascular devices, prosthetic heart valves, intravascular stents and pacemakers to the much larger total artificial heart. Whereas the artificial heart is still in the experimental stage, prosthetic heart valves, intracoronary stents and arterial grafts are in use worldwide. Knowledge of postimplantation change(s) and the cause(s) of failure is therefore critical.

#### 9.7.2.1   Prosthetic Heart Valves

Heart valve prostheses have been successfully implanted since 1960. That decade will probably be remembered by cardiologists as the decade in which heart valve replacement became a success story (Roberts, 1976). Over 50 different prosthetic heart valves had been introduced in the preceding 30 or so years. Many had to be discarded, and those that remained have gone through many modifications and continue to go through experimental studies towards modification. Generically, prosthetic heart valves are divided into mechanical and tissue valves. The basic principle in both types is 'passive moment', the pressure gradient deciding the opening and closure of the device, i.e. the response to pressure and flow changes in the chambers above and below the prosthesis is responsible for its opening and closure. Virtually all of these valves have a plastic/metal frame covered with cloth,

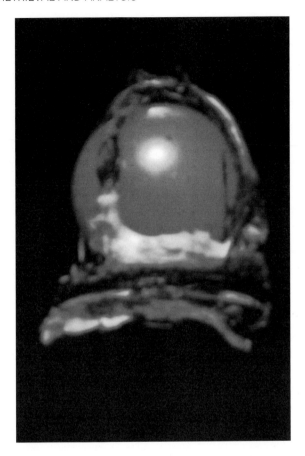

**Figure 9.7** A Starr–Edwards mechanical heart valve prosthesis removed after > 16 years' implantation. The sewing ring seen at the bottom of the illustration has largely been lost due to the surgical procedure, the cloth of the ring becoming 'trapped' in the host tissue making it difficult to excise completely. The occluder or poppet seen sitting inside the cage was originally a shiny white colour. Following long usage it has become pale, somewhat translucent yellow because of significant lipid insudation from the bloodstream. In addition, the valve shows a thick layer of pale white collagen-rich connective tissue on the ring and the bases of the struts. This was present all around the valve ring and hampered complete movement of the occluder, thus making the valve incompetent and stenosed. In addition to this, the valve struts show tissue and thrombus deposited on them. Their presence suggests haemodynamic abnormalities and/or lack of compliance with anticoagulant therapy. A common complication is pieces of this thrombus breaking off and embolising to the brain (or other organs), giving rise to thromboemboli and resulting in stroke

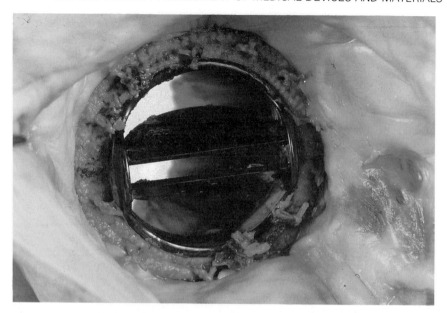

**Figure 9.8** A recently implanted St Jude Medical bileaflet medical prosthesis. The two hemispherical pyrolytic carbon discs are seen in the centre and the orifices on either side of the discs. This prosthesis was implanted in the mitral position

with the prosthesis itself being sewn into it; the cloth ring is used by the surgeon to sew the prosthesis in place.

### Mechanical Heart Valves

Such valves, manufactured of synthetic (non-physiologic) biomaterial, have a rigid but mobile occluder (ball or a disc(s)). Three major designs have been in widespread use, each one having three major structural components:

- base: the valve body or base on which the superstructure is mounted (Silver and Wilson, 1991)
- occluder: a rigid but mobile disc or poppet
- superstructure: a cage-like structure fixed to the base that guides and restricts the movement of the occluder.

Mechanical prosthesis currently in use worldwide include:

- Starr–Edwards caged ball valve (Figure 9.7)
- Bjork–Shiley (now Sorin Biomedical)
- Medtronic-Hall tilting disc valve
- St Jude medical bileaflet tilting disc valve (Figure 9.8).

The occluders of tilting disc and bileaflet valves are composed of pyrolytic carbon (Lilleihei-Kaster, OmniScience, Medtronic-Hall) or graphite coated with

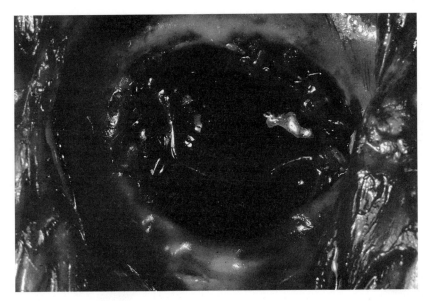

**Figure 9.9**  A Bjork–Shiley valve is seen in the mitral position. The prosthesis has been in place for several years and shows tissue growth on to the cloth-covered valve ring. In addition, there is soft thrombus on the valve ring and extending into the valve orifice. Running across the middle of the valve is the large inflow strut. The struts (outflow and inflow) hold the pryolytic carbon-covered tilting disc of the Bjork–Shiley valve in place. The presence of this thrombus on the atrial (flow surface) led to prosthesis dysfunction owing to incomplete opening and closure of the disc. In these cases, part of the thrombus should be taken for microbiological studies and histologic sections stained for microorganisms

pyrolytic carbon (Duromedics, St Jude medical bileaflet). The mechanical valve superstructures are made of pure titanium (Medtronic-Hall) or cobalt–chromium alloy (Starr–Edwards and Bjork–Shiley). In some cases the occluders and superstructure are both made of pyrolytic carbon (St Jude medical bileaflet). Blood flowing through a mechanical prosthesis has to pass around the occluder and its support, and hence areas of relative stasis are often unavoidable. These patients must therefore be maintained on lifelong anticoagulant therapy.

Several complications have been observed with the use of mechanical heart valves. A thrombosis rate of *ca.* 0.1–0.5% per patient year has been observed for such valves. Major factors leading to thrombosis are inadequate anticoagulant therapy and mitral positioning (Figure 9.9).

In patients receiving adequate anticoagulation the incidence of mechanical heart valve thrombosis is similar for caged ball, single disc and bileaflet tilting disc valves (Butchart, 1992). Clinically, the effects of valve thrombosis may be manifested slowly and progressively. Prosthetic valve thrombosis leads to valve dysfunction, i.e. incomplete opening and closure. Left-sided prostheses lead to pulmonary congestion, poor peripheral perfusion and systemic thromboembolism.

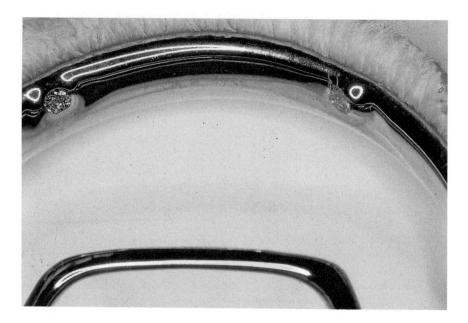

(a)

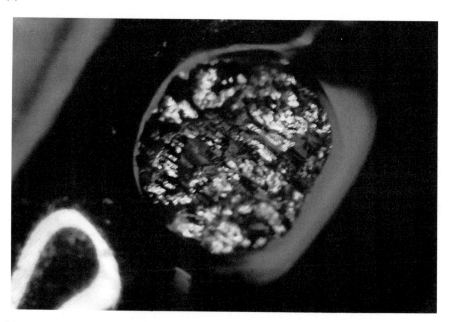

(b)

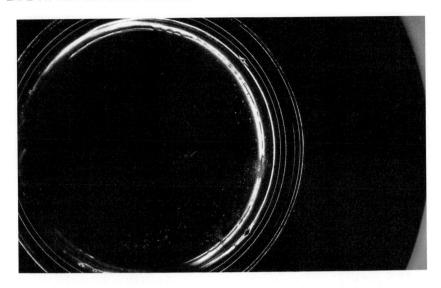

**(c)**

**Figure 9.10** These three photographs illustrate a Bjork–Shiley valve which has undergone structural failure. (a) Fracture of two legs of the small (outflow) strut. The leg on the left (of the illustration) probably fractured first, leading to friction between the two broken ends and smoothening of the fractured surfaces. The other leg probably fractured later. (b) A closer look at the left leg. (c) A close look at the disc of a Bjork–Shiley valve, which shows significant wear marks (the shiny ring) where the disc has been rubbing against the strut following fracture of the strut

Although the thrombosis may develop gradually, patients generally present with acute haemodynamic deterioration requiring immediate therapy. Echocardiography or fluoroscopy may both show a diminished movement of the disc or poppet. Prosthesis thrombosis has usually been treated surgically by explantation of the device and implantation of a new one. Today intravenous heparin therapy (thrombolysis) can be also used (Gueret *et al.*, 1995).

The incidence of major embolisation is *ca.* 4% per patient year in the absence of antithrombotic therapy, 2% per patient year with antiplatelet therapy and 1% per patient year with warfarin therapy. Most embolisation is manifested as cerebrovascular events (Edmonds, 1982; Burchfiel *et al.*, 1990). Thromboembolism is higher with mitral valve prostheses, caged ball valves and multiple prosthetic valves. In any patient with a prosthetic valve and embolisation, infective endocarditis and prosthesis thrombosis must be excluded.

Prosthetic valve infective endocarditis is relatively rare, but nonetheless a serious complication, being reported in 1–6% of patients. It is observed more in those who undergo valve replacement for infective endocarditis of their native valves. Theoretically, the incidence of infective endocarditis of mechanical heart valves and bioprostheses should be essentially the same. In both cases, an annular

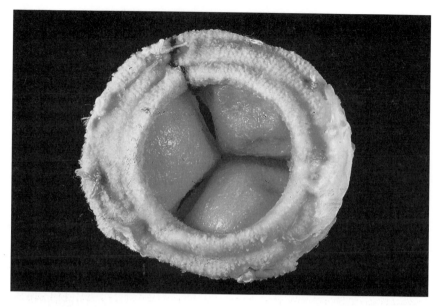

(a)

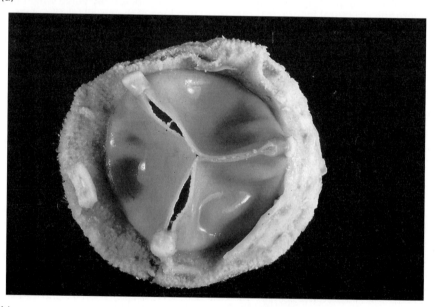

(b)

**Figure 9.11**   These figures show a bioprosthesis. (a) The flow surface of a Ionescu–Shiley bioprosthesis composed of bovine pericardium. (b) A non-flow surface of the bovine pericardial bioprosthesis. The three pericardial cusps are well seen. They are sewn in place, Dacron fabric mounted on a plastic frame being the sewing ring. At the stent posts (the vertical portions of the prosthesis) the adjacent cusps are held in place by a suture (the alignment suture). This prosthesis had excellent haemodynamics and a larger effective orifice area than a porcine bioprosthesis. However, tissue degeneration, largely related to abrasion

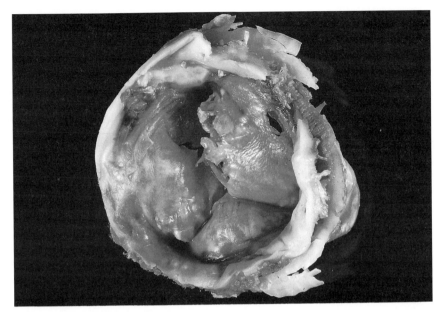

(c)

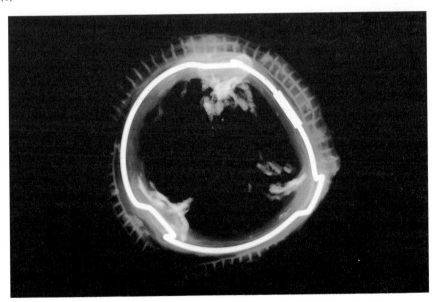

(d)

with the Dacron cloth and the alignment suture, led to early failure. The prosthesis has subsequently been taken off the market.

(c) and (d) These figures illustrate a porcine bioprosthesis. (c) A porcine bioprosthesis explanted several years after implantation, with extensive calcification of cuspal tissues and prolapse of two cusps (related to the calcification and cusp tears). The cuspal tissue is pale yellow in colour when the valve is fresh. (d) X-ray of a porcine bioprosthesis with significant calcification, much of it in the cusps at the commissural regions. The calcification extends into the adjacent porcine aortic root.

abscess may develop, i.e. infection of the tissues surrounding the prosthesis. In reality, however, it is far more common with mechanical valves. In bioprosthesis, infection often occurs on or around the cusps themselves.

Mechanical heart valves function well and for long periods without significant structural change. However, durability varies significantly among each category and between specific types of each (Jones *et al.*, 1990; Grunkemeier *et al.*, 1994; Yakob *et al.*, 1995; O'Brien *et al.*, 1995). Structural failure or fractures of contemporary mechanical tilting disc valves have been reported in a cluster of the widely used Bjork–Shiley (60° and 70°) convex-o-concave (C-C) prosthetic heart valves (Birkmeyer *et al.*, 1992; van der Graf *et al.*, 1992) (Figure 9.10).

In these, the weld points anchoring the two legs of the metal outlet (small) strut have fractured because of metal fatigue, leading to separation of the strut from the base, with secondary escape of the disc. The appearance of the fractured strut surfaces suggests that one strut fractures earlier and that disc embolisation results when both struts fracture. Separation of only one strut may occasionally be seen in an explanted valve. The Bjork–Shiley tilting disc (60° and 70°) has been taken off the market. However, disc fractures have also been reported with some bileaflet tilting disc valves, e.g. Duromedics (Klepteko, 1989).

### Bioprosthetic Heart Valves

Bioprosthetic valves are flexible and, to date, invariably trileaflet in design, so that they appear grossly identical to, and function in a manner akin to, natural cardiac aortic valves. These are usually comprised of animal (porcine or bovine) tissue (occasionally human) fabricated by chemical treatment, usually aldehyde cross-linking, and mounted on a stent or frame. Such tissue valves usually do not need anticoagulant therapy.

These prostheses may be (Cokouchoukos *et al.*, 1978):

- heterografts/xenografts (porcine aortic valves or cusp tissue derived from bovine pericardium)
- homografts/allografts (human aortic or pulmonary valves, generally from human cadavers and the recipient's heart following allograft heart transplantation; usually cryopreserved, not cross-linked, and implanted directly into the aortic root, with no stent). This type of valve usually lacks a surface layer of viable endothelial or connective tissue cells at the time of implantation, but does have biological blood-contacting surfaces and a central orifice similar to that of native valves, associated with significant haemodynamic efficiency, diminished turbulence and a lower rate of thrombosis
- autografts, i.e. valves fashioned out of the patient's own tissues, e.g. fascia lata (no longer used), pericardium or pulmonary valve (transplanted to the aortic position).

More detailed descriptions of bioprosthetic heart valves are available elsewhere (Schoen, 1991).

**Table 9.1** Prosthetic heart valves in common use

| Type | |
| --- | --- |
| **Mechanical** | |
| Caged ball | Starr–Edwards |
| Tilting disc | Medtronic–Hall |
| | Omnicarbon |
| | (Bjork–Shiley)[1] |
| Bileaflet | St Jude Medical |
| | Carbomedics |
| | (Edwards–Duromedics)[2] |
| | |
| **Bioprosthetic** | |
| Porcine | Hancock |
| | Hancock MO |
| | Hancock intact |
| | Carpentier–Edwards |
| | Carpentier–Edwards-SAV |
| Pericardial | Carpentier–Edwards |
| | Ionescu–Shiley[3] |
| Stentless porcine valves | T-SPV (St Jude Medical)[4] |
| | Hancock |
| | Carpentier–Edwards |
| Homografts | Cryopreserved aortic valves |
| | Fresh pulmonary valves |

[1] Now called the Sorin Valve (not sold in the USA)
[1-3] No longer in use. Explantation continues
[4] Canada and Europe. US clinical trials only

A recent modification of porcine aortic valves is the stentless porcine valve fixed with glutaraldehyde (Butany and David, 1994; Delrizzo *et al.*, 1995). Its outer surface is usually wrapped with a single layer of Dacron to facilitate implantation. Its advantage is that there is no pressure gradient (created by the presence of the stent) and it has a larger effective orifice area available for blood flow. Haemodynamically these bioprostheses function very well. However, they have only been in use for a limited time (since *ca.* 1991) and long-term data are not yet available.

With bioprosthetic heart valves primary tissue failure is the major concern and cause of prosthesis dysfunction (Figure 9.11a,b). Structural degeneration of the aldehyde-preserved tissue leads to cusp calcification and stiffening, with progressive stenosis of the orifice (Jones *et al.*, 1990; Grunkemeier *et al.*, 1994; Yakob *et al.*, 1995; O'Brien *et al.*, 1995) (Figure 9.11c,d).

Cusp tears may occur, with or without associated calcification, and lead to cusp prolapse and prosthesis incompetence (Figure 9.12).

Acute bioprosthesis failure is rare, but has been reported. It is related to sudden large tears of cuspal tissue. Among bioprostheses, the haemodynamically excellent and initially very well accepted first-generation pericardial bioprosthesis (e.g. the Ionescu–Shiley pericardial valve) showed early and significant deterioration,

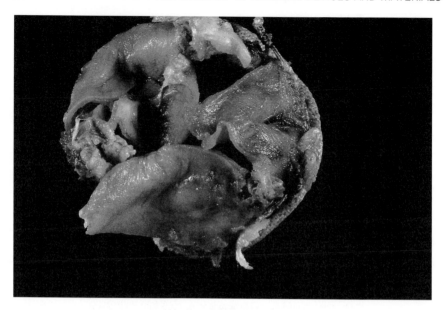

**Figure 9.12** This bioprosthesis, a Hancock pericardial valve, shows extensive tissue degeneration and cusp tears. All three of the cusps show tears at the stent post, extending down to the base of the cusps. All three cusps are prolapsed into the orifice. In some areas the posts show patchy grey-white tissue covering them, i.e. host tissue, pannus, which has grown on to the prosthesis. In addition, the three cusps have become thicker than usual, owing to insudation of tissue fluid, a fairly common finding in pericardial bioprostheses. In addition, the cusps show mild mineralisation. These changes led to severe prosthesis dysfunction and its explantation. The premature failure of this prosthesis was also related to abrasion damage

with significant cusp tears developing between 2 and 5 years postimplantation, mainly as a result of design failure, with abrasion-related damage. As a result this pericardial valve has been taken off the market (Figure 9.13) (Butany et al., 1992).

Long-term studies show that at 11 years prosthesis failure is virtually the same when mechanical valves are compared with biological ones. However, significantly larger numbers of mechanical heart valves function well at > 15 and > 20 years than do bioprostheses. At least 50% of porcine aortic valves implanted into mitral or aortic sites require replacement at 15 years postimplantation because of primary tissue failure. Regurgitation associated with cusp tear (usually associated with calcific nodules) is the commonest form of failure (Delorme et al., 1992; Turina et al., 1993). Cusp stenosis due to calcific cusp stiffening and cusp tears or perforation, without evidence of calcification, is less common, although the exception is probably the pericardial valve (Ionescu–Shiley and Hancock) described above (Butany et al., 1992).

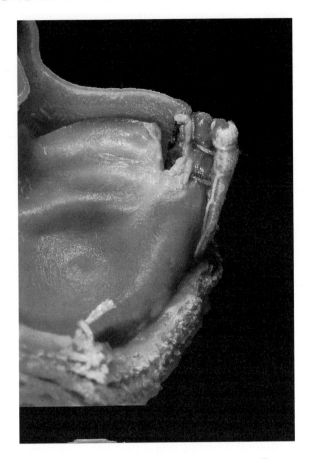

**Figure 9.13**  An Ionescu–Shiley pericardial bioprostheses. Two cusps are seen at the stent post. One cusp shows a nearly vertical tear (type 1 tear) close to the stent post and in the region where the alignment suture would have been located. These tears are related to abrasion damage to the biological tissues following constant abrasion against the Dacron cloth covering the prosthesis stent

### 9.7.2.2  Vascular Grafts

Vascular grafts are commonly used to bypass lesions in the vascular system. Large-diameter grafts are placed in the aorta when bypassing an aneurysm or when placing a valved conduit in the pulmonary or aortic valve positions. Similar though smaller synthetic bypass grafts are commonly employed in the iliac and femoral arteries and for creating arteriovenous shunts in patients undergoing chronic haemodialysis (Delorme *et al.*, 1992).

At the time of explantation of such a graft (human or experimental animal) their exact type, location and dimensions should be noted. Of particular

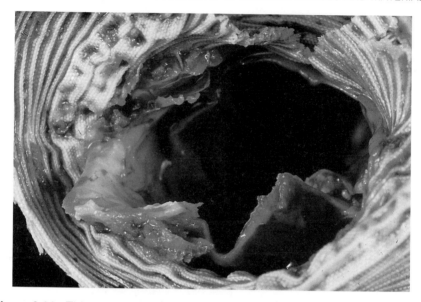

**Figure 9.14** This pleated Dacron graft was in place for more than 3 years. Its flow (inner) surface shows a thick layer of whitish brown tissue. This tissue is usually deposited at the proximal and distal ends of long grafts. This new intima may be lined by endothelial cells, and is then called the neointima

importance is the appearance of the graft (specifically its intactness), the presence of any thrombus formation (inside or outside the graft) and the presence of any tissue layer on the flow surface. The presence of any purulent-appearing material requires submission of a touch swab or piece of tissue for microbiological examination. At histological examination of the synthetic material and the tissue on either surface, cell morphology and the thickness of the ingrowth or deposited layers must be noted (Figure 9.14).

Histomorphologic and immunohistochemical analyses of the tissue growth on the inner aspect of the graft can also be performed to help decide whether tissue growth is pseudo- or neointima. Note must be made of tissue ingrowth (into the biomaterial) and the presence (and type) of cellular infiltrate in the weave of the fabric comprising the graft.

Long-term changes in vascular grafts can occur on both the outer and inner (flow) surfaces as well as in the graft material itself. The outer wall usually shows the formation of a fairly thick fibrous capsule. The junction between this capsule and the synthetic material itself often shows an infiltrate of mononuclear inflammatory cells, as well as multinucleated giant cells. These surround the fibres forming the synthetic graft. A similar outer capsule is seen around autologous vein grafts used for coronary artery bypass procedures. The inner or flow surface of prosthetic grafts tends to show a variable degree of fibrous tissue, at times admixed with thrombi deposited on the surface. At the point of junction

**Table 9.2**   Clinical characteristics of prosthetic valves

| Type | Profile | Durability | Thrombogenicity | Haemodynamics |
|---|---|---|---|---|
| **Caged ball** | High | Excellent | + + + | Fair |
| Single tilting disc | Low | Good to excellent | + + + | Fair |
| Bileaflet tilting disc | Low | Excellent | + + | Good |
| **Heterograft:** | — | Fair | − to + | |
| Porcine | — | | | Good |
| Pericardial | — | Poor–good[1] | − to + | Good |
| Stentless[2] | — | N/A[3] | − to + | Excellent |

[1] Poor for the Ionescu-Shiley
   Good, so far, for the Edwards pericardial
[2] For the aortic site only
[3] Not sufficient data to date

with the native vessel, significant tissue deposits may occur and lead to stenosis of this lumen. A false aneurysm may develop at the junction with the host vessel as a result of suture dehiscence and/or infection. This is an important complication, as it can rupture easily and lead to catastrophic bleeding.

Expanded polytetrafluoroethylene (PTFE) grafts (Gore-tex) function well for many years but, when used for arteriovenous shunts in patients on long-term haemodialysis, significant reaction to the material is observed at the sites of puncture. Fibrous tissue ingrowth into the graft, and a macrophage and multi-nucleate foreign body giant-cell reaction to the disrupted fibres is commonly found. Occasionally these areas undergo aneurysmal dilatation and necessitate removal of the graft (Tutassaura et al., 1978; Mohr and Smith, 1980). Commonly, however, such grafts last for several years and become dysfunctional through the development of a thick layer of tissue at the anastomosis, usually the venous end. This tissue is comprised of cells with morphological features of smooth muscle cells (stain positively for smooth muscle cell actin) with a collagen matrix.

### 9.7.2.3   Cardiac-Assist Devices

This category of cardiovascular device is composed of ventricular-assist devices (VAD) and artificial hearts. Both are still experimental, and an adequate and thorough analysis of explanted devices (after successful use or at autopsy) is even more critical. A standard format of evaluation should be used (Schoen et al., 1990). Both devices consists of pumps and valves connected to the patient's cardiovascular system.

### 9.7.2.4   VAD

As its name suggests, the VAD is a temporary device meant to assist one or the other side of the heart (usually the left). The objective of any study of clinically used VADs is to:

- document and characterise device changes, blood-contacting surfaces (smooth or textured), and the valves (tissue or prosthetic), conduits, compliance chambers, housing and other components (including energy packs)
- determine the cause of death or complications associated with device use. Perhaps the most common complication is valve thrombosis (despite anti-coagulant therapy) and infection.

### 9.7.3 ORTHOPAEDIC DEVICES

The handling of these devices has already been discussed. In cases where tissues are removed with the device, the membrane surrounding the implant often shows a diffuse discoloration. Histologically the surface shows granular, flaky, black material which does not stain with any of the routinely used dyes. These are predominantly extracellular metal particles, some of which may have been phagocytosed by histiocytes. Often, immunohistochemical investigation (using CD-68 markers) has shown the cells lining this capsule to possess the features of histiocytes. The quantity of foreign material and discoloration diminishes with distance from the implant (Amstulz, 1970).

Joint replacement arthroplasties and internal fixation devices for fractures (such as blades, screws, rods etc.) were originally made of stainless steel (Anderson, 1965) containing iron and significant quantities of chromium, nickel and molybdenum. Other metals used are titanium alloys, which contain aluminum and vanadium. Any of these elements can interact with tissues to form oxides (owing to electrochemical reactions and corrosion), resulting in the release, not only of the metals themselves, but also of the byproducts of interaction with the tissues. Eventually, following phagocytosis by macrophages, the elements can be carried to regional lymph nodes and other parts of the body. The presence of iron in tissue samples can be demonstrated by Perl's Prussian blue stain, whereas analytical TEM can be used to identify the individual materials and their location within the organelles of the cells. These are, however, time-consuming and expensive technologies and seldom used routinely.

In an effort to diminish the friction in an arthroplasty, some of the components have been replaced by plastic materials which articulate with any metallic components. Early arthroplasty cups were made of PTFE, but unfortunately these produced a significant foreign-body reaction (Charnley, 1961, 1970). The current generation of devices use ultrahigh molecular weight polyethylene (UHMWPE), but again this material has, with time, shown abrasion-related damage, leading to the release of microscopic particles into adjoining tissues. The body's response depends on the size and number of these particles and, in turn, determines the integrity of anchorage of the implant (Fornasier et al., 1991). Released particles from most polymers cannot be digested and are ultimately extruded from the cells, along with the enzymes present in the lysosome. A chemotactic reaction is then induced and more phagocytic cells appear: the phagocytosis cycle restarts and the foreign material will again be phagocytosed in an effort to break down the particles. Another cycle of inflammation occurs and the complete circle of events is maintained until the implant is loosened, causing pain and eventually necessitating implant replacement, with all its potential complications and costs. There is also ongoing research into the use of low-friction articulating surfaces such as ceramics (aluminium oxide) (Jaersho, 1981). Unfortunately, at this stage ceramics remain brittle and non-compliant compared to metals and polymers. The body's response to this material and its particles tends to be associated with a greater degree of membrane fibrosis. However, if the particles are released inside the synovium the reaction tends to be reduced, albeit still associated with peri-implant membrane enhancement.

## 9.7.4 BREAST PROSTHESES

Silicone is used in a very wide variety of medical devices, including intravenous tubing, pacemaker leads, orthopaedic prostheses (joint prostheses), replacement lenses, breast implants and many other items (Bush, 1994). Its chain length determines whether it is a liquid or a solid polymer. The most commonly used medical silicone polymer is siloxane, a major reason for its selection being its apparent biological inertness. Many studies have shown that silicone polymers contain many contaminants, e.g. fumed silica, platinum, low-MW polymers and other products (Bush, 1994). Whether or not some of these contaminants are chemically, physiologically and immunologically inert has still not been resolved (Autian, 1967). The recent high-profile legal and media attention devoted to breast implants has arisen as a result of the apparent medical problems/complications reported in women with silicone breast implants.

Breast implants (introduced in the 1960s) are used for cosmetic as well as reconstructive surgery following mastectomy for malignancy (Swan, 1994). Currently, there are three major types of breast implants available, namely saline filled, silicone gel filled and combination filled (gel and saline). The device consists of two components, the silicone polymer and the envelope in which it is contained. The implant's surface may be smooth or textured. The silicone used in breast implants is a major component of the silicone gel filler and a component of the implant covering or envelope. For cosmetic reasons the implants may be placed in the subglandular region, just behind the breast tissue, or in the subpectoral region deep to the pectoralis major muscle. In the latter location the device is much more deeply placed, and 40–60% of its surface is covered by the pectoral muscles. These devices, like any foreign material accidentally or intentionally placed in the human body, incite the same reaction. In all patients there is initial wound healing, resulting in a fibroblastic response and capsule formation. In the majority of recipients the prosthesis performs well and without significant complication. However, there have been many reports of 'side-effects' (Kumagi et al., 1984; Lazar and Lazar, 1991).

### 9.7.4.1 Special Characteristics of Silicone

An inert substance is one which, when implanted, does not incite a physiological reaction to itself, any degradation products or the physiological products released in the body's attempt to degrade it. Silicone, long believed to be inert, is apparently not so inert, if one accepts all the clinical and morphological complications attributed to it. In combination with enzymes and tissue proteins it can, and does (with or without another adjuvant), lead to an inflammatory response. Whether this response is to the silicone itself, the combination of silicone and the release of proteolytic enzymes when phagosomes/lysosomes rupture, or to the contaminants and other materials present in the silicone gel, is not certain. Nevertheless, a significant reaction is often observed (Kumagi *et al.*, 1984; Lazar and Lazar, 1991; Vasey, 1995). At this stage it is not certain how much of the silicone gel itself is actually metabolised or transported to other parts of the body over a significant period of years.

### 9.7.4.2 Silicone Bleed

Experiments over the last few years have shown that silicone is capable of leaving the site of implantation, especially when injected, and initiating a reaction (Kossovsky and Stassi, 1994). The early reaction is comprised of the appearance of polymorphonuclear leucocytes, plasma cells and macrophages. At a later stage lymphocytes, fibroblasts, plasma cells and macrophages are all found. This is associated with the formation of a fibrous capsule around the injected materials. In experimental animals it has been shown that, in addition to the formation of the fibrous tissue capsule, the implant site itself shows a significantly increased number of eosinophils, thereby suggesting possible immunological sensitisation to one or more components of the gel. The free injection of silicone into the peritoneal cavity in experimental animals has resulted in fibrous adhesions and histiocytic granulomas, a feature suggestive of chronic inflammation. The use of different batches of silicone gel has been shown to result in a variety of inflammatory responses as regards invasion by fibrous tissue, the severity of inflammation and the presence of multinucleate giant cells. It is quite possible, considering the spectrum of responses, that the observable changes are the result of impurities in the implanted material and not the silicone gel itself. These impurities include silica and platinum, the silica having been used to harden the elastomer silicone rubber (which comprises the capsule). Still other impurities include organic and inorganic compounds produced during the polymerisation process. Based on the evidence of Kossovsky and Stassi, it is at present difficult to make a case for any established cause-and-effect relationship, there also being other evidence suggesting no 'good' scientific proof to support the fact that silicone implants cause autoimmune symptoms (Schusterman *et al.*, 1993; Friedman, 1994).

### 9.7.4.3 Clinical Complications Associated with Breast Implants

In the vast majority of individuals these implants function well without inciting any significant response. The patients with significant untoward response are a minority and, in fact, the responses observed have been shown statistically to be similar in number to those that might have occurred had they not accepted breast implants; some plastic surgeons and rheumatologists have even gone so far as to suggest that sampling errors and media publicity have created a phantom disease. Among the common clinical problems reported in women with breast implants are joint pains, joint tenderness, lymphadenopathy, hair loss, sicca symptoms, dyspnoea, bladder dysfunction, connective tissue diseases and chronic fatigue syndrome (Vasey, 1995). On average, about 5 years after the implants have been placed, the breasts gradually become firmer (and may even become as hard as baseballs if calcified) (Redfern *et al.*, 1977). This is probably related to capsule formation and progressive capsular contracture. The progressive extension of the muscle, joint and nerve pains is believed to reflect the likely forward flow of silicone particles through the fascial planes and along the lymphatics following silicone bleed (Wintsch *et al.*, 1978). Obviously, therefore, this flow could ultimately involve the heart and lungs. In a recent study comparing the incidence of connective tissue diseases, e.g. rheumatoid disease, lupus etc., in women with and without breast implants, there was no statistical difference between the cases and the controls (Naaim and Lanzafam, 1993). In a different study, the same conclusion was arrived at, namely that there was no relationship between silicone breast implants and rheumatic disease (Gabriel *et al.*, 1994; Gabriel *et al.*, 1995; Salvarani *et al.*, 1995). However, in the latter case there was no study of the chronic fatigue/fibromyalgia syndrome typically found in symptomatic women with implants.

### 9.7.4.4 Pathological Findings in Breast Implants

The most common feature found in completely excised breast implants is a varying thickness and degree of fibrous tissue reaction to the implant. Histological examination shows that the capsule is comprised of collagen, with scattered foreign-body giant cells, possible granulomas, lipogranulomas and refractile foreign material, which may be intracellular or extracellular. The fibrous capsule itself may have histiocytes, and some of these may be foamy and contain lipid or lipid-like materials. The finding of chronic inflammatory cells is variable, as is the degree or severity of inflammatory infiltrate. If the surgeon has removed the regional lymph nodes, detailed examination of these may show granulomas containing refractile foreign material. Examination of the prosthetic implant must include examination of the surface, looking for intactness of the elastomer bag and the seal area, again for the same reason. The manufacturer's name and serial number may often be found on the area of the seal on the deep surface of the implant (Kossovsky and Stassi, 1994).

Silicone breast implants have been causally linked to local inflammatory and fibrotic reactions. They have also been associated with a number of autoimmune diseases, although this link is tenuous and debatable. Much of this local and systemic reaction has been attributed to impurities in the silicone gel and/or the capsule, which include silicates, polymerisation or partial polymerisation products, as well as the bleed and migration of silicone itself. It is reported that the systemic effects and autoimmune diseases may result from prolonged implantation of these devices. However, there is at present no definitive evidence to support this statement.

## 9.8 CONCLUSIONS

Today, numerous highly useful and often life-saving prosthetic devices are implanted by surgeons and physicians. Virtually all of these incite some reaction, usually primarily a mild inflammatory response and the deposition of a fibrous capsule. A small percentage of prosthetic devices are associated with some long-term complications, which may on occasion be life threatening. The most common of these is infection and this often necessitates removal of the device and its replacement with another. In other prostheses durability continues to be a problem. Detailed studies and ongoing and systematic examination of explanted devices is crucial to a better understanding of their mechanisms of failure and the development of newer, safer and more durable devices.

## 9.9 REFERENCES

Amstulz LIC (1970) Complications of total hip replacement. Clin Orthop 72:123–130.
Anderson ID (1965) Compression plate fixation and the effect of different types of internal fixation on fracture healing. J Bone Joint Surg 47A:91.
Andrews JN (1996) Cellular behaviour to injected silicone: a preliminary report. Plast Reconstruct Surg 38:581–583.
Ashley FL, Braley S and Reese TD (1967) The present status of silicone fluid in soft tissue augmentation. Plast Reconstruct Surg 39:411–420.
Autian J (1967) Toxicologic aspects of implants. J Biomed Mater Res 1:433–440.
Bienz K and Egger D (1995) Immunocytochemistry and in-situ hybridisation in the electron microscope: combined application in the study of virus infected cells. Histochem Cell Biol 103(5):325–338.
Birkmeyer JD, Marrin CAS and O'Connor GT (1992) Should patients with Bjork–Shiley valves undergo prophylactic replacement? Lancet 340:520–523.
Brett J and Kukatsu A (1995) Interaction of antibody with Forssman antigen in guinea pigs: a mechanism of adaptation to antibody and complement mediated injury. Am J Pathol 146:1260–1272.
Burchfiel CM, Hammermeister KE and Krause-Steinraufh (1990) Left atrial dimensions and risk of systemic embolism in patients with a prosthetic heart valve. J Am Coll Cardiol 15:32–41.
Bush H (1994) Silicone toxicology. Semin Arth Rheum 24:11–17.

Butany J, D'amati G, Fornasier VLF, Silver MD and Sanders GE (1990) Detailed examination of complete bioprosthetic heart valves. ASAIO Trans 36(3):M414–417.

Butany J, Vanlerberghe K and Silver MD (1992) Morphologic findings and causes of failure in 24 explanted Ionescu–Shiley low profile pericardial heart valves. Hum Pathol 23:1224–1233.

Butany J and David TE (1994) Pathology of explanted stentless porcine valves (human experience). In: Gabey S and Freighter RWM (eds) New horizons and the future of heart valve bioprostheses. Silent Partners Inc., USA.

Butchart EG (1992) Thrombosis, embolism and bleeding. In: Bodnar E and Freighter R (eds) Replacement cardiac valves. McGraw-Hill, New York, USA.

Charnley J (1961) Arthoplasty of the hip: a new operation. Lancet 1:1129.

Charnley J (1970) Acrylic cement in orthopaedic surgery. Churchill Livingstone, Edinburgh.

Cocke WM and Sampson HW (1987) Silicone bleed associated with double-lumen breast prostheses. Ann Plast Surg 18:524–526.

Cokouchoukos NE, Davila-Roman VG and Spray TL (1978) Replacement of the aortic root with a pulmonary autograft in children and young adults with aortic valve disease. Circulation 58:76–78.

Cotran RS (1993) Endothelial cells. In: Kelley WN (ed.) Textbook of rheumatology, 4th edn, WB Saunders Co, Philadelphia, USA.

Cotran RS, Kumar V and Robbins SL (eds) (1994) Inflammation and repair.In: Robbins SL (ed) Pathologic basis of disease, 5th edn. WB Saunders Co, Philadelphia, USA.

Davies PF and Tripathi S (1993) Mechanical stress mechanisms in cells: an endothelial paradigm. Circ Res 72:239.

Delorme JM, Guidoin R, Canizales S and Charara J (1992) Vascular access for hemodialysis: pathologic features of surgically excised PTFE grafts. Ann Vasc Surg 6:517–524.

Delrizzo DF, Goldman BS and David TE (1995) Aortic valve replacement with a stentless porcine bioprosthesis: a multicentre trial. Can J Cardiol 11:597–603.

Edmonds LH (1982) Thromboembolic complications of current cardiac valve prosthesis. Ann Thorac Surg 34:96–106.

Eichmeller S, Stephenson PA and Paus R (1996) The new method for double immuno-labelling with primary antibodies from identical species. J Immunol Meth 190(2):255–265.

Falk RH, Mackinnon J, Wainscoat J, Melikian V and Bignell AHC (1979) Intravascular haemolysis after valve replacement: comparative study between Starr–Edwards (ball valve) and Bjork–Shiley (disc valve) prostheses. Thorax 34:746–748.

Ferrans VJ and Butany J, Trump BF and Jones RT (eds) (1983) Ultrastructural pathology of the heart. In: Trump BF and Jones RT (eds), Diagnostic electron microscopy. Wiley & Sons, New York, USA.

Fornasier VLF, Wright JS and Seligman J (1991) The histomorphologic and morphometric study of symptomatic hip arthroplasty: a post mortem study. Clin Orthop 271:272–278.

Fornasier VLF and Cameron HU (eds) (1994) The pathology of prosthetic implants. In: Bone implant interface, Mosby Yearbook, Chicago, USA.

Friedman RJ (1994) Silicone breast prosthesis implantation and explantation. Semin Arth Rheumat 24(S1):8–10.

Gabriel SE, Ofalin WM, Kurland LT et al. (1994) Risk of connective tissue diseases and other disorders after breast implantation. N Engl J Med 330:1697–1702.

Gabriel SE, Ofalin WM, Kurland LT and Milton LJ (1995) Risk of connective tissue disorders (CTDs) among women with breast implants (letter). Life Sci 57:1737–1740.

Greenhalgh DG (1996) The role of growth factors in wound healing. J Trauma 41:159–167.

Grunkemeier GL, Jameson WRE, Millar DC and Starr A (1994) Actuarial vs actual risk of porcine structural valve deterioration. J Thorac Cardiovasc Surg 108:709–718.

Gueret P, Vignon P and Fournier P (1995) Transeosophageal echocardiography for the diagnosis and management of nonobstructive thrombosis of mechanical mitral valve prostheses. Circulation 91:103–110.

Hammermeister KE, Sethi GK, Henderson WG *et al.* (1993) A comparison of outcomes in men 11 years after heart valve replacement with a mechanical heart valve or bioprosthesis. N Engl J Med 328:1289–1296.

Jaersho M (1981) Calcium phosphate ceramics as hard tissue prosthetics. Clin Orthop 181:259–265.

Jensen HE, Schonheyder HC, Hotchi M and Kaufman L (1996) Diagnosis of systemic mycoses by specific immunohistochemical tests. APMIS 104(4):241–258.

Jones EL, Weintraub WS and Kraver JN (1990) Ten year experience with a porcine bioprosthetic valve: inter-relationship of valve survival and patient survival in 1050 valve replacements. Ann Thorac Surg 49:370–384.

Klepteko W (1989) Leaflet fracture in Edwards–Duramedics bileaflet valve. J Thorac Cardiovasc Surg 97:90–94.

Kossovsky N and Stassi J (1994) A pathophysiological examination of the biophysics and bioreactivity of silicone breast implants. Semin Arth Rheum 24(S1):18–21.

Kumagi Y, Shiokawa Y and Medsgerta (1984) Clinical spectrum of connective tissue disease after cosmetic surgery. Arthr Rheum 27:1–12.

Lazar AP and Lazar P (1991) Localised morphia after silicone gel breast implantation: more evidence for a cause and effect relationship. Arch Dermatol 127:263.

Lingenmayer TF (1992) Collagen. In: Hay E (ed.) Cell biology of the extracellular matrix, 2nd edn, Plenum Press, New York, USA.

McGrath MH and Burkhardt BR (1984) The safety and efficacy of breast implants for augmentation mammoplasty. Plast Reconstr Surg 74:550–560.

Metzdorff MT, Grunkemeier GL, Pinson CW and Starr A (1984) Thrombosis of mechanical cardiac valves: a qualitative comparison of the silastic ball valve and the tilting disc valve. J Am Coll Cardiol 4:50–53.

Mohr LL and Smith LL (1980) Polytetrafluorethylene graft aneurysms: a report of 5 aneurysms. Arch Surg 115:1467–1470.

Moore PJ (1995) Advances in immunoelectron microscopy. Meth Cell Biol 48:45.

Moreira JE, Reese TS and Kachar B (1996) Freeze-substitution as a preparative technique for immunoelectron microscopy: evaluation by atomic force microscopy. Micro Res Tech 33:251.

Naaim JO and Lanzafam CJ (1993) The adjuvant effect of silicone gel on antibody formation in rats. Immunol Invest 22:151–161.

O'Brien MF, Stafford EG and Gardiner MAH (1995) Allograft aortic valve replacement: long-term follow up. Ann Thorac Surg 60:S65–70.

Ratner BD (1983) Surface characterisation of biomaterials by electron microscopy for chemical analysis. Ann Biomed Eng 11:313.

Redfern AB, Ryan JJ and Su CT (1977) Calcification of the fibrous capsule about mammary implants. Plast Reconstr Surg 59:249–251.

Roberts WC (1976) Choosing a substitute cardiac valve, type, size, surgeon. Am J Cardiol 38:633–638.

Salvarani C, Gabriel SE, Ofalin WM and Hunder GG (1995) Epidemiology of polymyalgia rhematica in Olmsted County Minnesota 1970–71. Arth Rheumat 38:369–373.

Scheen FJ (1991) Pathology of bioprostheses and other tissue heart valve replacements. In: Silver MD (ed.) Cardiovascular pathology, 2nd edn, Churchill Livingstone, New York, USA.

Schoen FJ (1995) Approach to the analysis of cardiac valve prostheses as surgical pathology or autopsy specimens. Cardiovasc Pathol 4:241–255.

Schoen FJ, Anderson JM and Didisheim P (1990) Ventricular assist device (VAD) pathology analyses: guidelines for clinical studies. J Appl Biomat 1:49–56.

Schusterman MA, Kroll SS and Reece GP (1993) Incidence of autoimmune disease in patients after breast reconstruction with silicone gel implants *vs* autogenous tissue: a preliminary report. Ann Plast Surg 31:1–6.

Sheild PW, Perkins G and Wright RG (1996) Immunocytochemical staining of cytologic specimens: how helpful is it? Am J Clin Pathol 105(2):139–162.

Silver MD and Wilson GJ (1991) Pathology of mechanical heart valve prostheses and vascular grafts made of artificial materials. In: Silver MD (ed.) Cardiovascular pathology, 2nd edn, Churchill Livingstone, New York, USA.

Skoularigis J, Essop MR, Skudicky D, Middlemost SJ and Sareli P (1993) Frequency and severity of intravascular haemolysis after left-sided cardiac valve replacement with Medtronic-Hall and St Jude Medical prostheses and influence of prosthetic type, position, size and number. Am J Cardiol 71:587–591.

Snyderman R and Uhuig RJ (1992) Chemoattractants stimulus–response coupling. In: Gallin JJ (ed.) Inflammation: basic principles in clinical correlates, 2nd edn. Raven Press, New York, USA.

Swan SH (1994) Epidemiology of silicone-related disease. Semin Arth Rheumat 24(S1):38–43.

Thomas R and Lipsky PE (1993) Monocytes and macrophages. In: Kelly WN (ed.) Textbook of rheumatology, 4th edn. WB Saunders Co, Philadelphia, USA.

Turina J, Hess ON, Turina M and Krayenbuehl HP (1993) Cardiac bioprostheses in the 1990s. Circulation 88:775–781.

Tutassaura H, Gerein AN and Sladen JG (1978) True aneurysms in prosthetic femoral popliteal grafts. Am Surg: 262–266.

Valdre G, Mongiorgyi R, Monti S *et al.* (1995) X-ray powder defraction (XRD) in the study of biomaterials used in dentistry. Minerva Stomatologica 44:21–32.

van der Graf Y, de Waard S, van Herwerden LA and Defauw J (1992) Risk of strut fracture of Bjork–Shiley valve. Lancet 33:257–261.

Vasey FB (1995) Observations on women with breast implants. J Florida MA 82:348–351.

Wintsch W, Smahel J and Clodius L (1978) Local and regional lymph node response to ruptured gel filled mammary prosthesis. Br J Plast Surg 31:349–352.

Wright I (1992) Complement receptors and the biology of phagocytosis. In: Gallin JJ (ed.) Inflammation: basic principles and clinical correlates, 2nd edn. Raven Press, New York, USA.

Yakob M, Rasme SMI and Sundt TM (1995) 14 year experience with homovital homografts for aortic valve replacement. J Thorac Cariovasc Surg 110:186–194.

# 10
# Assessment of Biological Safety – Risk Analysis

JEREMY TINKLER
Medical Devices Agency, Department of Health, London, UK

## 10.1 INTRODUCTION

To take action without being absolutely certain of the result carries the risk that the outcome will not be as intended. Any intervention in the health status of a patient carries an unavoidable risk of an undesirable result, because the patient is already at risk from the prevailing medical condition and treatment is undertaken specifically to reduce that risk. Furthermore, uncertainty exists in our knowledge of physiological, pathological and therapeutic processes, and there is variability in any practitioner's choice of therapy, the skill with which it is applied and the patient's response to it. However, just as we learn to manage uncertainty in all aspects of our daily lives, we need to develop a mechanism to deal in the most effective way possible with this imperfect knowledge about the provision of healthcare.

Risks arising from the application of health technology have long been managed in some way, e.g. through the intervention of regulatory bodies (as has been the case for many years for medicinal products) or healthcare workers in accordance with their professional judgement and codes of practice. The introduction of the 'new approach' Directives to regulate medical devices throughout Europe places much of the responsibility for the control of device-related risks in the hands of manufacturers and Notified Bodies. This chapter is primarily intended to provide guidance for manufacturers on what should go into a toxicological risk analysis, so that the identified risks can be assessed in terms of the suitability of the materials for use in a particular product.

Risk management is not a perfect science: it has its own associated risks. There is always a risk that the measures taken to control risks will not prove adequate in practice. The result of this can be an adverse incident, with severe consequences both to patients and to the manufacturer. Litigation in the USA has sought to deny that uncertainty has a place in healthcare, such that injury is seen as the result of fault, rather than misadventure, and that liability must therefore follow.

*Biocompatibility Assessment of Medical Devices and Materials.*
Edited by Julian Braybrook. © 1997 John Wiley & Sons Ltd.

The consequences of this approach have been to the detriment of both the healthcare industry and healthcare providers worldwide, and thus ultimately to the detriment of patients. These consequences have included massive liabilities, the withdrawal of products and materials from the healthcare market and uncertainties about supplies and product quality. The fact that the most significant legal actions have been in response to concerns about biological safety highlights the importance of this aspect of conformity assessment during the development of new products.

To reduce the risk of these sorts of consequences, a risk management strategy needs to be adopted. It is foolhardy to ignore the hazards or take a gamble without knowing the odds. Instead, a rational course of action should be determined on the basis of a comprehensive assessment of the risks. Potential hazards need to be identified, the chances of them occurring and their probable consequences need to be analysed, and the uncertainty inherent in the analysis taken into account. This sort of analysis is the basis of sound risk management. Not only can adopting a strategy like this reduce the chances of an adverse situation occurring, it can also significantly reduce the severity of the consequences when one does occur.

It is neither practical nor desirable to reduce risks by the overzealous application of safety measures. A careful balance must be struck so that the risks identified can be controlled in a way which achieves the desired degree of safety without introducing further risks, e.g. by increasing the cost of a product to a level that restricts the activities of its user. It is important for the general improvement of public health that development costs must be contained within reasonable limits. In controlling toxicological risks the aim cannot be to achieve absolute safety: nothing is absolutely safe, and no material can be guaranteed to be fully biocompatible. Rather, the aim should be for a realistic level of assurance that the toxicity of the material has been adequately controlled. To achieve this aim, many complex factors need to be balanced. In some cases this will require a good deal of data, testing and expense. In other cases virtually no effort is required. By adopting an approach based on risk management, unnecessary testing and expense can be eliminated wherever possible, thus conserving valuable resources and achieving an appropriate level of safety assurance. It is fortunate that the methodology for such an approach is well established and readily adaptable to this situation. By analysing biological risks in a systematic way, a balanced approach is possible that can place known risks in a realistic context, thereby reliably and cost-effectively minimising the perils of adverse biological effects, defective devices and litigation.

## 10.2   REGULATION AND THE MANAGEMENT OF RISK

The imposition of legal controls affecting the activities of manufacturers, healthcare workers and the public is a form of risk management. Risk management involves applying a set of measures relevant to a particular set of significant risks and intended to restrict and maintain those risks within tolerable limits at a proportionate cost (Health and Safety Executive, HSE, 1995). Before tackling the subject of risk analysis as it relates to biological safety evaluation, it is necessary to review some of the basic principles of risk management that have been well established over many years, and to note how they have been applied to the field of medical device regulation. There are some differences in the way risk assessment is treated in different fields, but for the most part the same principles are followed in the management of industrial, environmental and healthcare risks. For medical devices, the principles are defined by the regulations by which they are controlled and by relevant standards, which can be an integral support for the regulatory system.

It does not matter whether control is achieved by direct intervention by government bodies, as in the USA and Japan, or through intermediaries, as is the case in Europe: the principles are the same. In the European Economic Area the regulations are provided by the medical devices Directives, which specify that risks must be acceptable when weighed against the intended benefits. European standards, which can be used to demonstrate conformity with the Directives and which address either the process of risk analysis or specific ways by which safety can be demonstrated, have been put in place. Regulations in the USA tend to be more prescriptive in terms of solutions to particular safety issues, but achieve the same risk management aims. Japanese regulations borrow extensively from standardisation, giving many of the control measures set out in international standards a regulatory status. In many other countries outside Europe there is a move towards the European model of 'light touch' regulation, based upon well-defined procedures for risk analysis and a balance between risks and benefits.

As a direct result of the emphasis that the European Directives place on assessing the acceptability of risk, CEN was directed to develop a standard on risk analysis. The European Commission and the relevant CEN Sector Board felt that clear guidance on how risks should be analysed was essential for the uniform and unambiguous verification of conformity with the Directives. A CEN WG began work in 1992 to review the established concepts of risk management and arrive at a consensus on how risk assessment should be handled in the conformity assessment of medical devices. The result of this work was the current European standard (EN 1441, 1997).

During their discussions, the CEN WG made extensive use of Guide 51 (now CEN/CENELEC Memo. No. 9) (ISO/IEC, 1990) which provides guidance on the inclusion of safety aspects in standards. Although this document is not particularly informative regarding risk assessment, it does provide the specific concepts and definitions upon which standards for medical devices have been based. Little has been written to date specifically on the management of the biological safety of medical devices; the increased prominence of the subject and the emphasis being placed upon it by regulatory bodies, e.g. the EC, has, however, created a demand for guidance in this area which is only now being met (Medical Devices Agency,

MDA, 1997; Tinkler, in press). Looking at the subject from a purely regulatory viewpoint, several other reference documents are available; they do not have specific relevance to medical devices but they provide general guidance on risk assessment and share a common understanding of regulatory aspects of risk control or toxicology (National Research Council, 1983; HSE, 1987, 1995; HM Treasury, 1991).

## 10.3  PRINCIPLES OF RISK MANAGEMENT

### 10.3.1  INTRODUCTION

The widespread application of the same techniques of risk management over a wide range of business and regulatory activities inevitably means that, with the different sorts of risks that are investigated, there will be differences in the way that risk assessment principles are implemented. A review of some of the basic principles of risk analysis, set out for example in EN 1441, will highlight the similarities and differences between the approach adopted for medical devices and that apparent in other areas of safety assurance.

### 10.3.2  HAZARD AND TOXICOLOGICAL HAZARD

A hazard is defined by EN 1441 and by ISO/IEC Guide 51 as 'a potential source of harm', where harm is any 'physical injury and/or damage to health or property'. There is no practical difference here from the definition used for industrial risk assessment, of 'the disposition of a thing, a condition or a situation to produce injury' (HSE, 1995). Injury can include harm, damage, adverse effect or detriment, i.e. 'the quantum of adverse consequences involved or presumed to be involved in the realisation of a hazard'. Hazard can be conveniently seen as a measure of some inherent property of a material or device, which can, in certain circumstances, lead to an undesirable effect. In identifying hazards related to medical devices, the investigation should not be limited to those giving rise to harm to health; the potential for adverse effects on the operations of a business or the cost of a product can be investigated in a similar manner, and they too can be detrimental to human health, in its widest sense. It is, in any case, unrealistic to expect that, in the development or marketing of a product, a manufacturer can divorce safety assessment from business decisions.

The biological safety assessment of medical devices is based on the principles of toxicology expounded by Philippus Paracelsus (1493–1541). He noted that all materials are poisons at a sufficiently high dose. It is important to remember that all medical devices, the materials from which they are made and all ingredients, additives and processing aids associated with those materials, pose some sort of toxicological hazard. Toxicological hazards are investigated by 'classic' toxicology studies, as opposed to some of the 'biocompatibility' tests routinely carried out on medical devices. These 'classic' studies investigate various aspects of the toxicity of a test substance at a range of doses, to obtain information about the nature of toxic effects and the dosages at which they occur, or at which no effect is seen. The concept of toxicological hazard takes into account the fact that some materials are more toxic than others in respect of the severity of the adverse effects that can be caused and the dose required to elicit those effects. The hazard is thus a property of the compound itself, rather than of exposure to it. A highly toxic material inside a closed container is no less hazardous because it has been safely contained.

## 10.3.3   RISK AND TOXICOLOGICAL RISK

At its most simple, risk can be defined as the possibility of more than one outcome occurring from a given set of circumstances (HM Treasury, 1991). In most areas of risk management, e.g. the insurance industry, risk is understood as the chance of something adverse happening, i.e. it is the mathematical probability of a particular hazard occurring. A more precise definition is 'the likelihood of a specified undesired event occurring within a specified period or in specified circumstances' (HSE, 1987). Here, the nature of the hazard defines the detrimental effect of the consequence, but does not affect the risk itself.

There are a number of areas where the probability of an occurrence is not considered sufficiently descriptive of the nature of the risk, and further specification of the risk, in terms of its characteristics, is necessary. This is particularly the case where people who are not in a position to make accurate risk calculations need to take account of residual risks associated with a hazardous activity. In the healthcare setting, practitioners need to be able to make assumptions about the risks inherent in the therapeutic measures they employ so that they can balance them against the benefits of the proposed course of treatment for an individual patient. In these circumstances, a low probability of a major hazard may be of equal value to a high probability of a minor hazard. The risk assessment therefore needs to take account of both the probability of occurrence and the severity of the hazard. This is reflected in the definition of risk given in ISO/IEC Guide 51 and EN 1441 as 'the probable rate of occurrence of a hazard causing harm and the degree of severity of the harm'.

A further concept to be included in our understanding of risk is that of 'uncertainty'. With increasing uncertainty, the probability of a correct prediction of outcome diminishes and, consequently, the risk increases. The HSE discussion document (HSE, 1995) notes that risk implies action in the face of uncertainty, and suggests that uncertainty is a 'felt deficiency in knowledge relevant to forthcoming decisions of critical importance'. Another way of looking at uncertainty (HM Treasury, 1991) is that it refers to the situation where the outcome of an action is open to doubt, or where the probabilities are unknown. This is in contrast to the concept of risk, in which the aim is to know the probabilities. In practice, it is often convenient and useful in risk management to consider risk and uncertainty as synonymous.

The reduction of uncertainty, in one form or another, is a means to effective risk assessment. Uncertainty is a particularly important factor in toxicological risk analysis, which relies heavily on extrapolation from experimental data. There are well-defined methods for dealing with this sort of uncertainty, e.g. those described in ISO Committee Draft (CD) 14538 (ISO, 1996b). With medical device materials, where experimental methods for biological risk assessment are generally of poor predictive value, uncertainty can be reduced by obtaining as many relevant data as is practical, from which a prediction can be made about biological safety in the intended application.

The probability that an adverse effect will arise from exposure to a chemical depends on the inherent toxicity of that chemical (the hazard) and the amount of it to which the subject is exposed, which in turn is influenced by the route of exposure. In its simplest form, therefore, toxicological risk is a function of toxicity and dose.

## 10.3.4   RISK MANAGEMENT AND CONTROL

'Risk control', although often used synonymously with 'risk management', can be more specifically applied to the sort of action taken by various professionals in identifying, limiting or managing risk. This includes carrying out risk assessments and making decisions related to safety. These activities may involve reducing risks or mitigating their consequences, or simply monitoring them to ensure that they are maintained at a level proportional to costs and benefits, or in line with identified priorities.

Many of the activities associated with medical device regulations are themselves examples of risk management. Included in these are the operation of a quality management system, which should encompass effective control of design, definition of product characteristics relevant to safety, verification that safety characteristics have been achieved during manufacture, responsible decision making in marketing, and the implementation of corrective action where necessary. Effective control of risks arising from the use of medical devices results in risks being reduced to an acceptable or tolerable level. Risks remaining after such measures have been taken are termed 'residual risks'. In the design of a device there is a need to reach a compromise between performance, safety and technical constraints. In striking such a balance it is inevitable that in some cases the residual risks will be substantial, but they must be balanced by anticipated benefits and mitigated by provision for corrective action (e.g. advice on dealing with adverse reactions or publication of advisory notices).

## 10.3.5   RISK ANALYSIS AND ASSESSMENT

Risk assessment is an essential part of risk management, and comprises a systematic process by which risks are estimated and equated with benefits so that a favourable balance can be demonstrated. Looked at in terms of a reduction of uncertainty, risk assessment can be seen as a way of increasing the chance of a successful prediction of outcome by improving the available information.

The collection and review of safety information and the consequent estimation of risk is termed 'risk analysis', and it is this aspect that is the subject of the standard EN 1441.

### 10.3.6   EN 1441

The requirements of EN 1441 are brief and straightforward, but act only as a general framework. The standard requires a structured procedure for risk analysis to be followed and documented. Information on relevant qualitative and quantitative characteristics must be collected and, from this, potential sources of harm (hazards) identified. The likelihood of harm arising from each hazard (i.e. the risk) can then be estimated, taking into account the severity of the harm. When all the identified hazards have been evaluated, the risk analysis needs to be documented so that a decision can be taken as to whether the apparent risks are acceptable. The acceptability of any risk varies with the intended application of the device, and will usually be assessed in relation to levels of risk known to be encountered in comparable situations. Acceptability also varies with time, and the continued validity of the risk analysis must be reviewed periodically in the light of new information and changing circumstances. The standard illustrates this procedure in the form of a flowchart, which is shown in Figure 10.1.

Although the scope of the standard is limited to risk analysis, it inevitably strays into the area of risk assessment. This is particularly the case when biological safety is investigated, as in this field it is virtually impossible to analyse risks without actually carrying out value judgements, which should strictly be classified as assessment. Furthermore, some of the information used in a biological safety assessment is itself the result of previous risk assessments.

The next few sections describe a procedure for conducting a toxicological risk assessment for a medical device material. As far as possible, the procedure follows the risk analysis method set out in EN 1441, and is consistent with the principles of risk control that are the basis of the European Directives for medical devices. As each part of the biological safety assessment process is explained its correlation with the EN 1441 procedure will be highlighted. Figure 10.1, which shows the procedure specified by EN 1441, should be referred to as a reminder of the identity of and interrelation between each step.

## 10.4   BIOLOGICAL SAFETY ASSESSMENT PROCEDURES

### 10.4.1   INTRODUCTION

Biological safety assessment combines aspects of risk analysis, assessment and control. Unfortunately, it does not always combine them in a conveniently logical

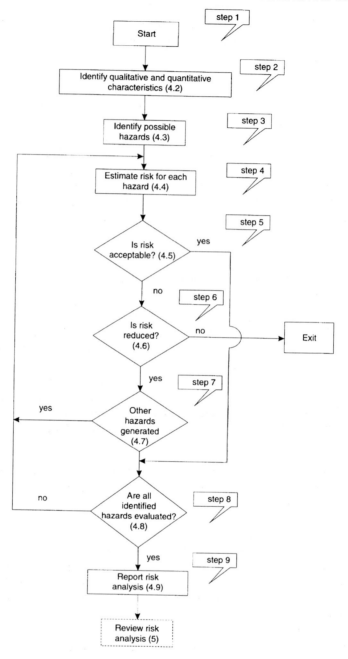

**Figure 10.1**   Flow diagram representing the risk analysis procedure

sequence. This is not a problem in practice, except when it comes to explaining, in a textbook, the theoretical basis of biological safety assessment, in terms of an established risk analysis model.

In line with EN 1441, the aim of a biological safety assessment is to identify any biological hazards arising from the materials used in a medical device and to investigate the resultant risk posed by its proposed use. It is inevitable that the process of biological safety assessment does not fit the EN 1441 procedure precisely. Elements of risk assessment or control creep into the risk analysis section, and it is common practice to cycle between analysis and assessment, collecting more information each time, until it can be concluded that the risks have been adequately controlled. Biological safety assessment is strictly a risk management tool, rather than a risk analysis method. It is as well to think of it as embracing entirely the principles of EN 1441, without necessarily following the sequence of its requirements.

## 10.4.2  TOXICOLOGICAL RISK ASSESSMENT

It is not possible to identify precisely what information may be needed for a biological safety assessment in any given set of circumstances, as because the aim is simply to reduce the overall level of uncertainty to a workable level, the lack of one particular type of data may be compensated for by analysis of another type of data. In general, biological safety data are required in respect of all components of a device with tissue, blood, mucous membrane or fluid path contact. The three basic types of information required for a toxicological risk analysis are identified in an Annex to EN 1441 and in the UK Competent Authority guidance on biological safety assessment (MDA, 1996) as well as in ISO 10993-1. These are:

- materials characterisation
  Toxicological hazards are a property of the chemical composition of a material. Data relating to formulations, residue levels, degradation products, effects of processing etc., allow the chemical identity of the material(s) to be fully characterised and the toxicological hazards identified.
- information on prior use
  Well established and documented clinical use of materials or their chemical components in an analogous situation is often the principal indication of their suitability for the intended purpose. Risks anticipated to arise from the intended use are assumed to be similar to those known to be clinically acceptable in the comparable situation.
- toxicological data
  Data from basic toxicological studies provide information on the hazards associated with the test materials employed in the studies. This information must be interpreted in the light of material characterisation data, which provide an estimate of exposure to the hazard. Biological tests which use representative samples or extracts of finished product as the test material usually provide

information directly on risks, rather than on hazards. Although such tests tend to be difficult to quantify, acceptable results give some degree of reassurance that the risk of adverse reactions occurring during clinical use is low.

These data types will be examined in more detail in the following sections. The data and analyses referred to represent an essential element of design control, as specified by an ISO 9001 quality system. They should be contained in, or referenced by, a design dossier or device master record. They need to be available for review by a regulatory agency or Notified Body, and the latter should be expected to review such data routinely.

## 10.5   MATERIALS CHARACTERISATION

### 10.5.1   INTRODUCTION

Information on the composition of a medical device material is crucial to any biological risk analysis because the hazards we are interested in are due to the chemical nature of the materials to which the body is exposed. Of the three data elements introduced above, it is often the most easily quantified, accurate, comprehensive and informative. These are the very qualities of data that are important in the reduction of uncertainty, and hence of risk. A biological risk analysis based on materials characterisation gives a good return for the invested effort and should be given a high priority.

The thought of carrying out a systematic characterisation of the chemical composition of a medical device tends to throw many people into confusion and panic. Collecting the necessary data is often perceived as an onerous task. It is true that, in some cases, it can be complex and time consuming. Usually, however, sufficient data are already available to a manufacturer or can be obtained quite easily. There is a critical distinction between information that is necessary and information that can be omitted or for which substitutes can be adopted. It is necessary to recognise the significance of the data available in order to identify any deficiencies in those data and to find suitable ways of rectifying such deficiencies.

Remembering that toxicological risk can be considered to be a product of both toxicity and dose, quantitative data on chemical composition are used to provide the dose element of this equation. Equating these data with available information on the toxicity of each identified component allows a systematic review of toxicological risks. In practical terms, the first step in the toxicological risk analysis is to itemise the chemical components of a material (including additives, processing aids and contaminants) and consider potential reaction or breakdown products. The logical starting point for this is the material formulation. A knowledge of the chemical processes occurring during manufacture can then indicate which components have the potential to be present in the final product. Ideally, quantitative formulations for each material with tissue or fluid path contact should be available. This may be considered good practice in all cases, but complete quantitative formulations are rarely essential. The requirement is to obtain sufficient data about the identity and availability of chemicals in the device to enable a risk assessment to be carried out. In some cases, i.e. where the presence of significant toxicological hazards is likely, this will require quantitative data on formulations or residues. Where this is the case, the argument that an identified risk was not assessed because quantitative chemical data were not available is seldom, if ever, valid. The greater uncertainty inherent in biological data rarely allows them to substitute adequately for quantitative chemical data.

Equating the biological safety assessment process with the steps set out in EN 1441 presents a few complications, as there is rarely a convenient differentiation between risks and hazards. Although toxicity is an inherent quality of a material (and thus a hazard), it is a relative concept and thus has a quantitative component: some materials are more hazardous than others. As already noted, dosage (or quantitative exposure data) can be considered an indicator of risk. Whereas the initial steps of EN 1441 deal exclusively with hazards in investigating the composition of a device, we are already investigating data that speak of risks. At each stage in the risk assessment process we need to make the best use of whatever data are available, whether quantitative or qualitative: it would not do to ignore available data simply because they do not fit in with the standard procedure.

The listing of potential components of a device is analogous to step 2 of EN 1441 (identification of qualitative and quantitative characteristics). The result is a list of materials or chemical compounds which could affect the safety of the device. If the materials characterisation data available are quantitative in nature, subsequent steps of EN 1441 can be carried out simultaneously.

EN 1441 requires that the risk arising from each identified component be analysed. At this stage in a biological safety assessment it is usual to depart slightly from the procedure outlined in EN 1441. Whereas it would be usual to proceed to step 3 (identification of possible hazards), it may be more practical either to go first to step 4 (estimation of risk for each hazard) and to return to step 3 later if necessary, or to consider steps 3 and 4 together. The actual procedure adopted in any circumstance depends on the nature of the information available.

## 10.5.2 IDENTIFICATION OF HAZARDS

Applying the requirements of step 3 of EN 1441 (compile a list of potential hazards), the list of chemical components should be reviewed and those which represent a potential toxic hazard identified. This presents something of a *non sequitur* in terms of toxicological theory, as all materials are toxic to some extent and are thus potentially hazardous. The risk of toxic effects arising is dependent on the dose. In practice, a distinction can be made between compounds that are of concern and those that are most unlikely to cause harm. A value judgement needs to be made by the toxicologist as to what constitutes a 'significant' hazard. Taking into account the available knowledge about the toxicity of the compound, including the potential for any synergistic effects, those compounds that would not be expected to lead to adverse effects at the maximum level of exposure conceivable from the intended use can be classified as 'non-hazardous' and discounted. Again we run into a problem of semantics, as this judgement requires information on both toxicity and expected dose: it is actually a risk assessment, rather than hazard identification (and thus completely outside the scope of EN 1441). Irrespective of this distinction, the net result of the rather sweeping assertion that certain chemicals are 'non-hazardous' is that most chemical constituents of a device can be excused any further consideration. Taking this concept to its logical conclusion, where materials characterisation reveals that a device can contain no 'hazards', there can be no risk and little further analysis is required. This represents a major short-cut in the risk assessment.

There is a difference between this approach and the 'generally regarded as safe' concept that has been used with foodstuffs. This concept is one that should always be approached with caution because it usually oversimplifies the situation. For medical devices, as with many other applications, the significance of a particular toxic hazard varies with the circumstances of exposure. In addition, the maximum conceivable level of exposure depends on device-related factors. It is thus a matter of experience and judgement whether a particular compound represents a potentially significant hazard or not when used in a particular device. If this were not so, it would be possible to publish an 'approved' list of materials which were certified as being suitable for use in all devices. Although many people ask for such a list, they must remain disappointed because such issues can only be decided on a case-by-case basis.

## 10.5.3  ESTIMATION OF RISKS

Where particular toxicological hazards are identified, the risk arising needs to be estimated from quantitative data. Armed with a knowledge of the chemical constituents of a material and their toxicity, it is necessary to estimate and determine the acceptability of the risks arising from the compounds that have been identified as potential hazards. The requirement of EN 1441 is, for each of the possible hazards identified, to estimate the risk in both normal and fault conditions using available information/data. Remembering that risk is a function of the toxicity of a compound and its availability, which are analogous to hazard and probability in our risk control model, risk estimation must comprise an analysis of quantitative data on the availability of each compound in the light of its toxicity. In this situation, toxicity can be defined as a combination of the ability of a material to cause harm to health, and the nature of that harm. Availability can be seen as the probability of the material reaching a site of action in the body where it can cause that harm. The risk estimation asks 'What is the likelihood of harm to health arising from this exposure?'.

In most cases, confirmation that a chemical or material does not present an undue risk is all that is required. The assessment of what constitutes an undue risk is another area for the exercise of judgement. There are no absolutes here. One cannot expect an entirely risk-free situation: one can only seek a degree of risk that is felt to be comfortably remote. This can be termed a 'tolerable' risk, which is one where the availability of a compound is such that harm to health is not expected to result. This is determined on the basis that hazardous chemical residues are not delivered to body tissues at a level likely to result in a toxic response.

Determining the availability of each constituent of a material would involve a large number of expensive toxicokinetic studies, which would make the development costs of even the simplest medical device prohibitive. Thankfully, this sort of analysis is rarely necessary. As has already been stressed, this phase of an investigation is only reached where potential hazards have been identified and a residual risk is suspected. Where further analysis is necessary, the use of worst-case assumptions allows a stepwise approach to the estimation of availability to be adopted. Quantitative data on formulations, residues, leaching, absorption or uptake by particular tissues provide a basis for a conclusion on availability. These types of data are listed here more or less in order of decreasing availability and increasing cost. It must be remembered that only sufficient data are required to indicate that the level of exposure is so low that the risk of toxicity is sufficiently remote. In the majority of cases data at the cheap and available end of the scale will suffice.

Careful control of polymerisation reactions can ensure that residues of toxic precursors are minimised. The combination of a knowledge of relevant chemistry with quality assurance information can provide sufficient reassurance in many situations. Where residues of toxic precursors, processing aids or reaction products do exist, many tend to be bound within the matrix of the device material. Again, a knowledge of chemistry will indicate whether leaching to a significant extent is a possibility. Where uncertainty remains, it will be necessary to carry out leaching studies. If sufficient safety assurance can be obtained, by assuming that all of the residue either present in or leached from a material is available at the site of biological action, it will not be necessary to measure absorption. This assumption is not only a reasonable worst-case scenario: for implanted devices it is realistic. Only where there is particular concern about toxic effects occurring in practice will more accurate estimates of tissue exposure be required.

Where materials have an extensive history of prior use it may not be necessary to investigate their individual chemical components: an assessment can be made on the basis of the suitability of the material as a whole. Requirements therefore differ between established and novel materials. It is necessary to investigate chemical composition in detail only for novel materials or for known materials with ingredients that present a significant toxicological hazard. All materials were novel at some stage, of course, and one might naively assume that they were thoroughly investigated at the time of their introduction.

Although it is possible to evaluate the suitability of a material without analysing its chemical composition, this is not recommended. The resultant risk analysis would be much less rigorous and therefore less certain. As uncertainty equates with risk, the risk is thereby increased. It can also be argued that conformance with EN 1441 cannot be claimed unless hazards are identified, and hazards can only be identified through chemical characterisation of the materials.

## 10.6    ANALYSIS OF DATA ON PREVIOUS CLINICAL USE

The clearest indication that a material is suitable for a particular use is given by reliable data showing satisfactory performance in analogous situations. This point is borne out by the Level 1 European standard for implants, EN 14630 (CEN, 1996) which gives equal weight to a material found suitable by proven clinical use in similar applications as to one found acceptable following a documented assessment in accordance with the principles of EN 30993-1. This reveals a typical misunderstanding of ISO 10993, in that it ignores the fact that a decision on suitability on the basis of prior use is encompassed within the standard, rather than being an alternative to it.

It is possible, and indeed common, to evaluate suitability primarily on the basis of prior use, but this always requires some knowledge of the identity of the material and thus some degree of material characterisation. In such cases, assurance is required that materials are comparable from one application to another. Sufficient detail must therefore be known about the materials to allow the assessor to determine equivalence. This may be limited to reliance on a trade name, backed up by a quality system or vendor agreement. It is important to note here that a biological safety assessment cannot be considered relevant outside the context of a quality management system through which verification is available that the materials used meet the design specification. As a result, the supplier's quality system can be just as important as that of the manufacturer.

Ideally, data from clinical investigations and post-market surveillance should provide an indication of biocompatibility, i.e. demonstrate a desirable biological interaction with the device. Unfortunately, available data on prior use very rarely take the form of relevant studies addressing material biocompatibility. Very few investigate the biological performance of a device in such detail, although the sort of intrusive investigation required to obtain these sorts of data could not normally be justified. Clinical evaluations can, however, confirm that no adverse reactions were apparent during a scientific study designed to identify problems. Furthermore, as indicated in the previous chapter, an accepted and widely utilised approach to explant retrieval and analysis for the purposes of providing additional data of the required detail should help to overcome this current lack of information for the future.

Further assurance can be obtained from a knowledge of the extent of prior use of a material and the number of reported adverse reactions, although some caution is necessary here. Very few adverse reactions to medical device materials (as opposed to adverse incidents with medical devices) are reported, either to manufacturers or to regulatory agencies. It is likely that this is because they are misinterpreted as reactions to drugs or accepted as a 'normal' anticipated side-effect, and not that they do not occur. It may also be that healthcare staff are unaware of the mechanisms by which adverse incidents should be reported, or of the need to report adverse reactions in the same way as mechanical failures. Whatever the reasons, the result is that a lack of reported incidents is no guarantee of a lack of adverse reactions.

In spite of the underreporting of adverse reactions, the main justification for using a particular material or ingredient remains that it has been used before in similar applications. It is not unreasonable to expect that the unsuitability of a material would be detected during clinical use which, after all, is monitored by experienced professionals. Although there is no evidence to guarantee this, it is generally recognised to be the case. More specifically, the European Directives are based firmly on the principle of 'state of the art', the acceptance of a material on the basis of prior use being an example of the operation of this principle.

In practical terms, then, what information is required to demonstrate favourable prior use? For many materials this can be quite straightforward. If comparable products can be identified, information on the number of units sold and the number of adverse reactions reported can be reviewed. Data from any clinical studies should also be assessed. Even when the material used previously is not identical, prior use data are valuable: many of the ingredients of a medical device material will have been used previously and the toxicological significance of chemical differences in materials between devices can be assessed. Quantitative changes in formulation can be assessed through a knowledge of formulation or residue data. Data on the previous uses of a compound in medical device materials and the concentrations at which it was included can be considered along with information on its toxicity and the results of biological tests using materials in which it has been used. This combination of data is often a very good indication that a material which is similar in terms of composition also presents a similar level of toxicological risk. The influence of a novel ingredient on the overall biological risk can be assessed from quantitative data on its availability in the final product, coupled with data on its toxicity.

## 10.7  ANALYSIS OF BIOLOGICAL TEST DATA

Just as the purpose of a clinical evaluation for CE marking purposes is to provide very basic safety and performance data for devices that have not been tried and tested in clinical use, the purpose of biological testing is to provide preliminary data for new biomaterials, prior to their use in humans. The tests routinely available are, for the most part, designed not to demonstrate biocompatibility, but to identify toxicity. To expect more than this from them is unrealistic. As a result, except prior to the first clinical use of a material, biological tests should not be used as a primary source of safety data. Instead, their role should be to provide confirmation that the risk of an adverse reaction in humans is remote, i.e. a sort of 'belt and braces' role, whereby biological tests are used to corroborate the results of the analysis of data on material composition and past use.

The reason for this apparent lack of confidence in biological test data is the general lack of sensitivity and specificity of the tests. There is no doubt that tests can provide useful information on the suitability of a material when used in their proper context, as a component of a systematic evaluation. Unfortunately, it appears that biological testing has been given undue prominence and importance over the past few years. The tests listed in ISO 10993-1 are safety assurance tests: even though they are often termed biocompatibility tests, they do not provide a detailed characterisation of the interaction between a material and its biological environment. It is increasingly apparent that biological safety is becoming a sensitive issue, and it is therefore bad practice to place greater reliance on testing than is justified by the conclusivity of the results.

Determining the need for biological testing is a risk assessment in itself, or, more precisely, a cost–benefit assessment. The benefit is measured in terms of the value of the information gained from the test: the more sensitive the test and the more indicative of the clinical situation, the more valuable it is. Cost can be measured both in financial terms and in terms of animal welfare. There is no virtue in carrying out a test when the costs outweigh the benefits. In fact, it is either stupid or unethical, and often both. Unfortunately, unwarranted testing is fairly common; regulations and ethical values about animal testing vary from country to country, and this has a marked effect on the cost–benefit balance. More surprisingly, ideas about the value of biological test data also appear to vary between countries. In fact, the only constant factor is that testing is universally expensive.

This variability makes drawing common guidelines very difficult, but some pointers can be given. First, the need for testing should be considered on a case-by-case basis, taking existing data into consideration. The benefit of a particular test should be assessed by asking what additional assurance the test will provide about the material. This will depend on whether the data already available address the risks investigated by the end-point of the test. If there are adequate data from other sources to allow a conclusion that the risk of sensitisation or mutagenicity, for example, is acceptably low, testing becomes superfluous. The benefit of a test also depends on its sensitivity. Irritation, sensitisation and systemic effects are all risks that are clearly relevant to many devices. Irritation and sensitisation tests are well established and can be readily interpreted to provide relevant information on the risks associated with the device. The acute systemic test, on the other hand, rarely provides meaningful data and its value tends to be lower in many circumstances. Bringing animal welfare into the picture raises two considerations:

- *in vitro* tests should be carried out before *in vivo* tests unless it is certain that *in vivo* tests will be required
- any *in vivo* study should be justified on the basis of scientific need.

In some countries, failure to observe this basic humanitarian code is illegal. Finally, where animal welfare is not an issue, financial cost can be used to influence testing strategy. Cytotoxicity testing (discussed in Chapter 6) does not use animals, is comparatively cheap and, although it is difficult to relate the results of the test to a specific clinical end-point, test methods are being developed to provide greater specificity. Most importantly, however, it is sensitive.

## 10.8  CONCLUSIONS

ISO 10993-1 defines the role of biological tests within a structured programme of evaluation, within which the need for testing must be considered on a case-by-case basis, in light of all the considerations outlined above. The standard requires that a justification be given, not only for the waiving of tests but also for the decision to perform a test. The manufacturer thus takes on the full responsibility for the scientific and ethical integrity of the evaluation programme. It is no longer acceptable to say that a test was carried out as it is a regulatory requirement, because regulations no longer have testing requirements, only requirements to evaluate safety. There can now be only one approach to biological safety assessment: one which is based on a reasoned and scientifically valid analysis of risks. This must attempt to reduce uncertainty in the most expedient way by making use of the most relevant and predictive data available. This is the most effective way of providing a suitable level of assurance that biological risks have been controlled within acceptable limits.

## 10.9  REFERENCES

CEN EN 14630 (1996) Non-active surgical implants – general requirements. CEN, Brussels, Belgium.
CEN EN 1441 (1997) Medical devices – risk analysis. CEN, Brussels, Belgium.
EC (1990) Council Directive 90/385/EEC concerning active implantable medical devices. L189(20 July):17-24, Official Journal of the European Commission, Brussels, Belgium.
EC (1993) Council Directive 93/42/EEC concerning medical devices. L169(12 July):1-43, Official Journal of the European Communities, Brussels, Belgium.
HSE (1987) The tolerability of risk from nuclear power stations. ISBN 0 11 883982 9 HMSO, London, UK.
HSE (1995) Generic terms and concepts in the assessment and regulation of industrial risks. HSE, Suffolk, UK.
HM Treasury (1991) Economic appraisal in central government – a technical guide for government departments. HMSO, London, UK.
ISO 10993-1 (1996a) Biological evaluation of medical devices, Part 1: Evaluation and testing. ISO, Geneva, Switzerland.
ISO/CD 14538 (1996b) Determination of allowable limits for residues in medical devices using health-based risk assessment. ISO, Geneva, Switzerland.
ISO/IEC Guide 51 (1990) Guidelines for the inclusion of safety aspects in standards. ISO, Geneva, Switzerland.

MDA (1997) Clinical investigation guidance note no.5. DH, London, UK.

National Research Council (1983) Risk assessment in the federal government: managing the process. National Academy Press, Washington DC, USA.

Tinkler JJB (in press) Biological safety and European medical device regulations. Quality First Intl. Ltd., London, UK.

# Index

*Index compiled by Geoffrey C. Jones*